I0407227

Diabetes Selfcare Management

A patient-empowerment manual

Sarah Cuschieri
Charles Savona-Ventura
[editors]

Malta
2022

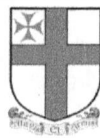

Diabetes Selfcare Management – A patient-empowerment manual
© Grand Priory of the Maltese Islands - MHOSLJ, Malta, 2022
Publisher: Lulu Press Inc, 627 Davis Drive, Suite 300, Morrisville, NC
27560
ISBN: 978-1-4709-4591-6

Contents

3

Preface

The Grand Priory of the Maltese Islands of the Military and Hospitaller Order of Saint Lazarus of Jerusalem embraced the principle of the Office of the Grand Hospitaller of the Order to help set up a Resource Library aiming at making available self-empowerment tools for individuals in need. These resources are available gratuitously online but can be purchased as hard-copy printed versions at publication costs.

This current self-empowerment targeting individuals with diabetics has been commissioned from professionals working closely in the field and having regular close contact with patients. Diabetes and associated adiposity has become a worldwide epidemic accounting for a high proportion of morbidity and mortality associated with chronic medical conditions.

This publication is a further welcomed self-empowerment resource in the Grand Hospitaller's Resource Library supplementing the previous publications produced by the Grand Priory of Canada – *A Caregiver's Guide* – *A Handbook about End-of-Life Care* available as a soft copy from the Grand Priory's website [1] and that produced by the Grand Priory of the Maltese Islands – *First Aid Manual* available as a soft copy from the Grand Priory's website. [2]

We do hope that these resources serve their purpose in addressing the primary aim of the Order's existence, that 'to assist, succour and help the poor, sick and the afflicted, especially those suffering from leprosy or similar diseases without distinction of religion, race, origin or age.'

---

[1] https://hospicetoronto.ca/PDF/Acaregivershandbook_CHPCA.pdf
[2] https://www.saintlazarusmalta.com/_files/ugd/
c2e348_e6ff3e8ff7634c7fa187edd369af9cb8.pdf

Introduction [1]

What is diabetes mellitus?

Diabetes is a worldwide disease affecting a large proportion of the world's population. In 2021, it was estimated that 5.1 billion adults (20 – 79 years), about 10.5%, were living with the disease. Reported statistics must be tempered with the knowledge that a large number of diabetic individuals are as yet undiagnosed or else are still in the pre-diabetes stage. [2] The prevalence of the disease has been steadily increasing over the last decades especially in affluent communities because of its association with obesity. Diabetes mellitus has a long history and has been described in antiquity, with the first complete clinical description being reported in the second half of the 2nd century A.D. by the Greek physician Aretaeus of Cappadocia.

Diabetes occurs when the body is unable to maintain a normal level of blood glucose (sugar). Glucose is the main source of energy of all the cells in the human body and thus is the main fuel driving the normal physiological functions of the body. Excess glucose goes to the liver to be stored as glycogen. Blood glucose levels are maintained in a healthy threshold by a regulatory system involving an interplay of hormones produced by the pancreas, insulin and glucagon, responding to amount of glucose available in the blood stream and the real-time energy requirements of the body. Insulin is the hormone which is responsible for the transport of blood glucose (originating from food and drink) into the body's cells. The glucose within the cells is then converted into energy or else stored for later use. Insulin also plays a role in the metabolism of protein and fat. Glucagon keeps blood glucose from dropping too low by stimulating the production and release of glucose from the liver cells thus ensuring that basic metabolic needs are maintained at sufficient levels to preserve life.

[1] Prepared by Dr. Sarah Cuschieri & Prof. Josanne Vassallo.
[2] International Diabetes Federation (IDF) Diabetes Atlas 2021 - 10th Edition

Diabetes occurs as a result of the body's inability to produce sufficient amounts of the hormone insulin needed by the body – insulin deficiency. Alternatively, another form of diabetes results from the inability of the body to effectively utilize the insulin produced by the body– insulin resistance. The hyperglycaemia associated with long standing undiagnosed or uncontrolled diabetes will result in long term complications, such as heart problems, stroke, eye disease, kidney damage, nerve damage etc. with detrimental effects on the individual's quality of life and even early death. In 2021, uncontrolled diabetes was responsible for an estimated 6.7 million deaths (1 death every 5 seconds).

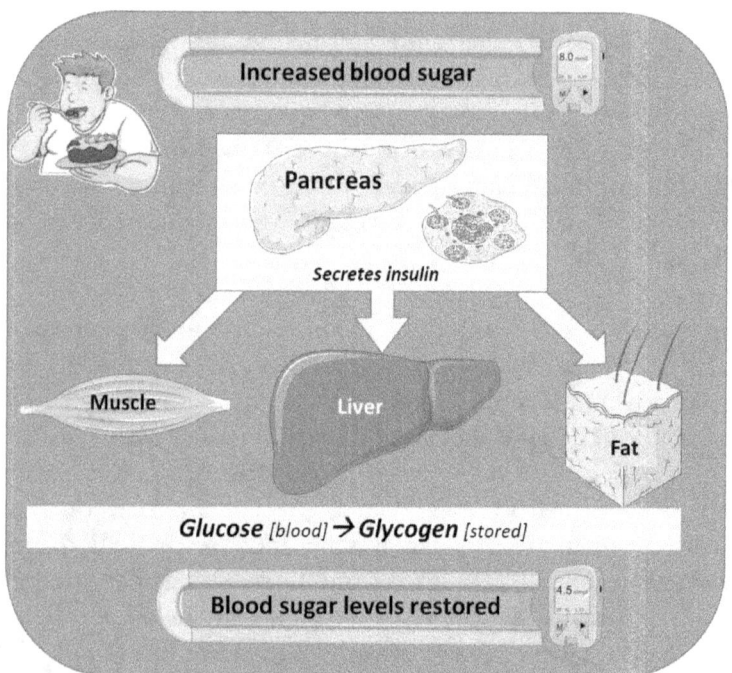

Physiology of blood glucose control

The impact of diabetes is not just restricted to the level of the individual, but has a significant effect at a public health level. The greater is the number of individuals with diabetes and resulting diabetic complications within the community, the greater is the burden is on the public healthcare systems as more people will require these health services (both on an outpatient and

8

inpatient basis). The total health expenditure due to diabetes in 2021 was estimated at US$966 billion being assumed to be on average two-fold higher than the expenditure for people without diabetes. Therefore, controlling diabetes and reducing/delaying the long-term complications associated with the condition, as well as preventing new onset diabetes, will have a positive impact not just on the quality of life of the individual but also on the economic healthcare sustainability of the country. The release of these funds from diabetes care issues would of course help provide resources to cover other healthcare needs of the community.

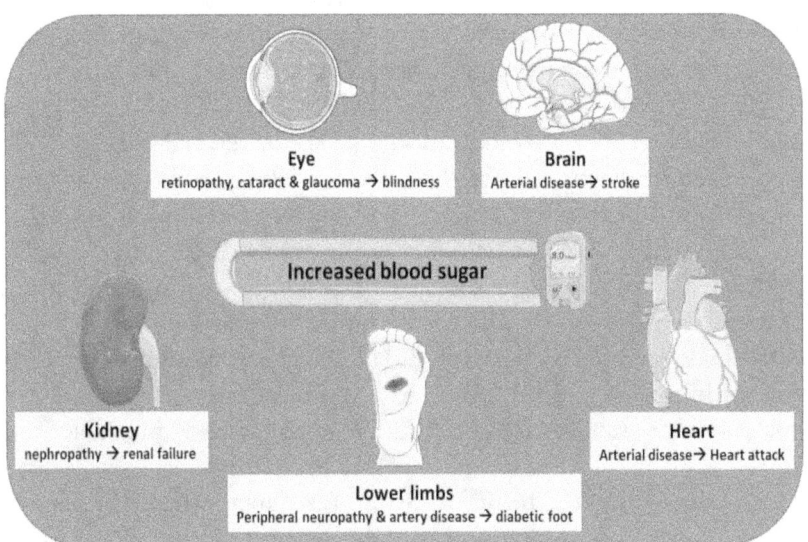

Long-term complications of uncontrolled diabetes

Classification of diabetes mellitus

Diabetes can be classified into different categories. Mention has already been made that diabetes could be the result of two potential mechanisms, that of relative or absolute insulin deficiency and that of insulin resistance by the cells of the body. These mechanisms acting alone or in tandem will give rise to various categories of diabetes mellitus.

i. *Type 1 diabetes* mostly occurs in children and young adults. It is the result of an autoimmune process where the immune system of the individual destroys the cells (beta cells) of the pancreas responsible for the

9

production of insulin. The condition would thus give rise to a situation of insulin deficiency. Individuals with type 1 diabetes would thus require daily insulin injections or an insulin pump to maintain a stable blood glucose level. The main predisposing risk factors for type 1 diabetes are genetic abnormalities and family history of type 1 diabetes. Viruses have also long been suspected to be involved in the development of type 1 diabetes, but consistent evidence connecting viruses to the condition has been hard to come by. The incidence of Type 1 diabetes varies from one population to another and is reported to range from 0.1-60.0 per 100,000 children aged 0-14 years.[1] Autoimmune forms of diabetes however have also been known to occur in adults when the condition is referred to as Latent Autoimmune Diabetes of the Adult or LADA.

ii. *Type 2 diabetes* is the most common type of diabetes. Although typically discovered or diagnosed in the mature adult from the age of 45 years onwards, it is becoming commoner at any stage of adulthood including in children and adolescents. This is the result of the growing obesity epidemic among the population which predisposes to the development of type 2 diabetes. It is estimated that globally about 462 million individuals are affected by type 2 diabetes, corresponding to 6.28% of the world's population. More than 1 million deaths were attributed to this condition, ranking it as the ninth leading cause of mortality.

Type 2 diabetes is the result of insulin resistance, which is the inability of the body's cells to respond to the circulating insulin. This prompts the production of more insulin resulting eventually in pancreatic cell failure. The same process of insulin resistance occurs in someone who is obese and hence, in these individuals, the persistent high demand made on the pancreatic cells over time will predispose that individual to developing diabetes.

The development of type 2 diabetes often occurs gradually through a two-stage process, although some individuals shift immediately from a state of normal glucose to full-blown diabetes. Those experiencing the two-stage process will initially develop prediabetes – often referred to as "borderline" diabetes in non medical terms. Prediabetes occurs when the glucose level is abnormally higher than normal but not high enough to qualify as type 2 diabetes. These individuals can revert to normal glucose stage following healthy lifestyle choices. Sometimes oral hypoglycaemic agents are also started during the prediabetes stage but lifestyle remains the mainstay of treatment. However, a number of individuals progress forward from prediabetes to type 2 diabetes, in which case the individual has a permanently high glucose level.

There are various risk factors contributing to type 2 diabetes. These can be broadly divided into preventable and non-preventable factors. The preventable risk factors include those factors that the individual can try to avoid. These include a sedentary lifestyle (little or no exercise), obesity, smoking, too much alcohol consumption, having a high blood pressure, and having high levels of "bad" fats in your blood. The non-preventable risk factors include factors such as being aged more than 45 years of age, having a family history of type 2 diabetes, having a history of gestational diabetes (see below), women having polycystic ovarian syndrome (PCOS), certain ethnicity races such as African Americas, Latino Hispanic Americans, Asian Americans, Pacific Islanders and Native Americans.

Maintaining a healthy lifestyle including following healthy dietary choices and physical activity is a key pillar in type 2 diabetes management plan. If this does not sufficiently control the blood glucose levels, then oral hypoglycaemic medication will be required. In some instances, if the glucose level remains high irrespective of being prescribed a combination of oral and injectable hypoglycaemic agents, the individual will need to be started on insulin injections.

iii. *Gestational diabetes* (GDM) is the occurrence of abnormal high glucose levels during pregnancy that does not persist after delivery of the baby (postpartum). This high glucose level is first diagnosed during pregnancy, typically in the last three months of pregnancy. The occurrence of GDM arise from as a result of the gradual increase in insulin resistance that is common as pregnancy progresses particularly in overweight and obese women combined with insufficient secretion of insulin to overcome the reduced action of insulin. There are various risk factors that can contribute to the development of GDM including a family history of diabetes, previous history of GDM, previous unexplained stillbirths, unhealthy diets, being overweight or obese, being above the age of 40 years and ethnicity race. The reported incidence of gestational diabetes varies from one community to another, but globally, GDM is estimated to affect about 15.0% of all pregnancies.

iv. *Monogenic diabetes* arises from a single gene abnormality (mutation) and can result in a broad spectrum of different monogenic diabetes forms. Maturity-Onset Diabetes of the Young (MODY) is one of the monogenic forms which typically presents at an early age (before 25 years) with raised blood glucose levels. This is characterised by impaired secretion of insulin.. There are many forms of MODY, all arising from a single gene abnormality and varying from very mild forms of diabetes treatable with diet and exercise to severe forms requiring blood glucose lowering medications. . Monogenic forms of diabetes are estimated to have an overall estimated prevalence of about 0.2 cases per 100,000 children and youths aged less than 18 years.

v. *Other specific types of diabetes:* Diabetes can occur following the occurrence of other pancreatic diseases such as pancreatitis (inflammation or infection of the pancreas), trauma to the pancreas, pancreatic cancer, and pancreatectomy (removal of the pancreas). Certain endocrinological disorders, such as Cushing's syndrome, can also lead to the development of diabetes; while some medications can disrupt the action of insulin or its secretion, resulting in a diabetic profile. For example the use of steroids to treat a number of other conditions often unmasks the tendency to diabetes. Additionally, some specific genetic syndromes, such as Down's syndrome and Prader-Willi syndrome, are also associated with diabetes.

Selfcare in the prevention and treatment of diabetes
Many individuals with abnormalities of blood glucose are as yet undiagnosed and thus live with persistently elevated blood glucose levels. The hyperglycaemic environment will initiate a gradual cascade of changes that will cause organ damage.

It is therefore essential that an early diagnosis is made so that timely management interventions can be instituted to slow down the adverse effects of hyperglycaemia. It is therefore very important that after the age of 45 years, when type 2 diabetes generally starts to develop, regular health check-ups are performed. Individuals who are at higher risk, such as those having a family history of diabetes or the obese or any other kind of chronic disease/s, should seek medical advice at a younger age. Women with diabetes during pregnancy are at increased risk of developing diabetes later in life and they should be counselled to undergo regular screening for diabetes.

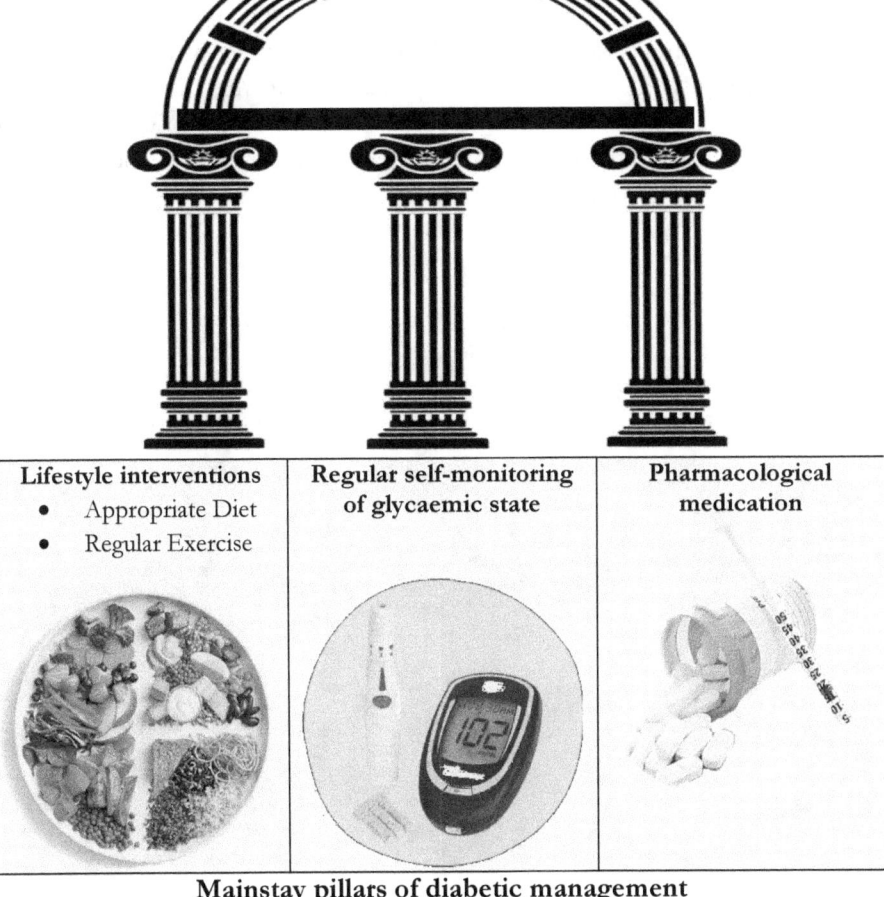

Lifestyle interventions	Regular self-monitoring of glycaemic state	Pharmacological medication
• Appropriate Diet • Regular Exercise		

Mainstay pillars of diabetic management

The primary pillars of the management regimens include lifestyle and medical interventions with appropriate pharmacological agents. This Following a healthy lifestyle including opting for healthy eating complemented by physical activity is an essential step in the selfcare regimen of diabetes. It is also essential that appropriate self monitoring is regularly performed by the individual in order to ensure close control of the glycaemic state. The anxiety and frustration that those living with diabetes experience as well as the sense of being at the mercy of their condition have been well documented and care of diabetes must of necessity include self care and mindfulness.

It is the aim of this booklet to introduce the principles of management to as wide a population as possible in appreciation of the various issues and challenges that those living with diabetes face on a day to day basis. We hope that by increasing awareness we can contribute to both the wellbeing and quality of life of those with diabetes.

Dietary control and weight management for diabetes prevention and intervention [1]

Introduction

In former times being diagnosed with diabetes meant that you had to radically change your diet and that the food experience is at the end! Nowadays, guidelines have been updated and emphasize on individualized dietary interventions that allow people to eat various foods based on personal preferences, culture and most important to fulfil personal nutritional needs and health goals. Indeed, there is no 'diabetes diet' but a diet that is based on individualized needs that can control blood sugar levels.

The causes of diabetes are multifactorial but there is much evidence showing that apart from non-modifiable risk factors such as genetics, age and ethnicity, modifiable factors such as diet and physical activity are integral part of self-management.[2] A group of researchers have shown that seven (7) essential self-care behaviours improve blood sugar control and reduce medical complications in people with diabetes, namely (a) risk-reduction behaviours, (b) effective problem-solving skills, (c) monitoring of blood sugar (d) complaint with medications (e) healthy coping skills (f) physical activity and (g) healthy eating.[3] The aim of this chapter is to briefly describe the basics on how components of the diet effect blood sugar levels highlighting the importance of weight control for diabetes prevention and management. The purpose is to give you a practical approach on how to improve dietary knowledge, attitude, and appropriate self-care that leads to better control of diabetes.

---

[1] Prepared by Dr. Mario Caruana Grech Perry & Dr. Claire Copperstone.
[2] Khazrai, Y.M., Defeudis, G. and Pozzilli, P. (2014) "Effect of diet on type 2 diabetes mellitus: A Review," Diabetes/Metabolism Research and Reviews, 30(S1), pp. 24–33. Available at: https://doi.org/10.1002/dmrr.2515
[3] Shrivastava, S.R.B.L., Shrivastava, P.S. and Ramasamy, J. (2013) "Role of self-care in management of diabetes mellitus," Journal of Diabetes & Metabolic Disorders, 12(1). Available at: https://doi.org/10.1186/2251-6581-12-14

The effect of food on diabetes

In countries that were directly involved during both World Wars, drops in diabetes death rates were recorded due to food shortage.[4] This clearly showed that dietary components have a direct effect on blood sugars. The human body breaks down food you eat and absorbs it in different parts that contain (a) carbohydrates; (b) proteins; (c) fats and (d) other nutrients including vitamins, minerals, alcohol, and other nutrients known as phytochemicals.

A) Carbohydrates

Fruit, starchy foods (such as cereals, bread, potatoes, pasta, and rice), sweet foods (biscuits, chocolate, sweets, jams), sugary drinks (juices and sweetened beverages) and milk and milk products all contain carbohydrates known as 'carbs'. When carbohydrates are digested, they are ultimately converted into glucose which is known as blood sugar. All types of carbohydrate will increase your blood sugar level. The more carbohydrates you eat, the greater will be the impact on blood sugar levels. It is thought that sugars (known as simple carbohydrates), such as table sugar (known as sucrose), cause a quicker spike in blood glucose levels than starches. However, gram for gram, sucrose and starch cause a similar blood glucose response when given in the context of a meal with a matching content of protein and fat (see section on Effect of Food). Carbohydrates in liquid form taken alone are absorbed quicker than those in solid food. Thus, having a sugary drink will produce a faster increase in your blood sugar levels than eating a slice of bread but a similar effect on blood sugar level is obtained if the carbohydrate content is similar. The table at the end of the chapter shows commonly consumed foods and drinks and the amount of carbohydrates they contain.

Dietary fibre is one constituent of carbohydrates that is not converted into blood sugar and can slow the absorption of carbohydrates. In fact, the general rule of thumb is that if food contains more or equal to five (5) grams of dietary fibre per serving (see section on reading the Food label),

---

[4] Lumey, L.H. and Van Poppel, F.W. (1994) "The Dutch famine of 1944-45: Mortality and morbidity in past and present generations," Social History of Medicine, 7(2), pp. 229–246. Available at: https://doi.org/10.1093/shm/7.2.229.

half of the dietary fibre is subtracted from the total grams of carbohydrates. The total is the actual carbohydrate amount that you should be considering. For instance, if food contains twelve (12) grams of carbohydrates and six (6) grams of fibre, the amount of carbohydrates that will affect your blood sugar is nine (9) grams (12 – ½ of 6). Hence, carbohydrates that contain fibre are preferred to highly processed carbohydrates as the former have a less impact on blood sugars and contain more nutrients than the latter.

The fibre content of food partly relates to the concept of glycaemic index (GI) known as 'low or high GI food'. GI is a term used to quantify how much a specific food containing carbohydrates will raise the blood glucose level. Nevertheless, there are other factors apart from fibre content that can influence the GI levels of these foods such as (a) processing (mashed potato has a higher GI than a baked potato), (b) ripeness (the riper the vegetable or fruit, the higher the GI value), (c) cooking technique (the time it takes to cook the food), and (d) variety (brown pasta and white pasta). A simple example can be given using oranges; if you drink orange juice, your blood sugar level increases quickly; if you take orange sauce, your blood sugar level increases a little more slowly; and if you eat a whole orange, your blood sugar goes up least of all.

To summarise even though carbohydrates raise your blood sugar levels, foods with carbohydrates should not be avoided. Being careful with the portion sizes and when possible, substituting with high fibre carbohydrates, is more important, especially if you are taking insulin. Carbohydrates provide you with energy (e.g., the brain uses carbs for energy) and contain important minerals, vitamins, and phytochemicals as those found in fruit. There are general guidelines as to how many carbohydrates you should eat but individualised recommendations are better suited as the amount needed depends on age, weight, physical activity, and state of health.[5] Monitoring the amount of carbohydrates is an integral part of diabetes management. It is now widely accepted that carbohydrates have the

---

[5] Davies, M.J. et al. (2022) "Management of hyperglycemia in type 2 diabetes, 2022. A consensus report by the American Diabetes Association (ADA) and the European Association for the Study of Diabetes (EASD)," Diabetes Care, 45(11), pp. 2753–2786. Available at: https://doi.org/10.2337/dci22-0034.

greatest effect on blood sugar levels. Although protein and fat do not contain carbohydrates, they may still indirectly contribute to diabetes.

B) Protein and fat

High protein foods include lean meats, chicken, fish, eggs, cheese, and nuts. These are an important part of the diet and on their own usually have minimal impact on blood sugar level. Yet, proteins can also provide energy and be turned into glucose if 'carbs' are not available. In fact, this is an important concept for people who are on insulin treatment as they need to increase insulin amount in relation to protein content of the meal. Protein can take anywhere from three (3) to four (4) hours to be digested, so a much slower rate than carbohydrates. It is important to note that protein foods usually also contain fats.

The other major nutrient in our food is fat, which is also needed by the body. Not all fat is the same, so eating specific types and controlling amount is key to weight management (see section on Health Eating). Like proteins, fat does not break down into glucose and has a minimal impact on blood sugar levels. Like fibre, fat may slow blood sugar breakdown and change the timing of the blood sugar peak after a meal. It can slow gastric emptying (the time is takes for food to go from the stomach to the small intestine) and may increase insulin resistance through weight gain. A higher-fat meal can affect post-meal blood sugar levels out of proportion to what you might expect based on the carbohydrates eaten, as the blood sugar peak is seen after many hours.

C) Other nutrients

Alcohol, in moderation, can be consumed for most people with diabetes. It may even contain phytochemicals that are beneficial for the body (e.g., wine), but the limitation is that alcohol can lower blood sugar levels, especially if on insulin or SGLT- 2 inhibitors. This is because as a nutrient, alcohol interferes with your blood sugar levels as alcohol reduces the capability of the body to make its own sugars from the liver. The key to moderation is for men with diabetes to restrain their alcohol intake to two (2) drinks per day and women one (1) drink per day, if there are no specific medical contraindications.[6] The size of the glass and type of alcohol affects the number of units, so it is best to check a guideline.[7] Avoidance of binge drinking is important and therefore the recommended one to two drinks per day cannot be saved and then taken all at once (binge).

There is scarcity of scientific proof regarding the benefits of vitamin supplements for people with diabetes who do not have a clinical vitamin deficiency. Vitamin supplements are only recommended for pregnant, breastfeeding, older adults, or vegan individuals. There is also a shortage of scientific verification regarding the benefits of food supplements that contain magnesium, chromium, and vitamin D to improve blood sugar control. Similarly, scientific evidence regarding the benefits of vitamins that work as antioxidants (vitamin C, vitamin E and beta-carotene) and omega-3 fats in diabetes is lacking.

There is research which is looking at other phytochemicals which are found in healthier food options (see section on Health Eating) and looking at their bioactive components which might have a significant lowering effect on blood sugar level and play a role in prevention of diabetes-related complications. While scientific evidence demonstrating the value of spices (cumin, curry, cinnamon, pepper, and ginger) that contain such phytochemicals to control blood sugar is missing, they are safe for most people who have diabetes. Regarding herbs, there is also no clear scientific proof that they can improve blood sugar levels. Although herbs are a good substitute to salt and increases palatability of food, it is always important to discuss any interaction with medications, especially with herbal supplements that exist in high concentrations.

D) Meal planning
As discussed in the previous sections, eating mixed meals is helpful in controlling blood sugar levels. Protein, fat, and fibre help delay the

---

[6] Diabetes UK (2022) Alcohol and diabetes Available at: https://www.diabetes.org.uk/guide-to- diabetes/enjoy-food/what-to-drink-with-diabetes/alcohol-and-diabetes Accessed 15th September 2022.
[7] The Sense Group (2022) Drink Aware Malta. Available at: https://www.drinkawaremalta.com/how-to-handle-alcohol/ Accessed September 2022.

digestion of carbohydrates which in turn reduces a sudden increase in blood sugar levels after meals. Therefore, meal planning and getting the right proportion of the required nutrients in the amount that your body needs is crucial in diabetes management.

Meal planning is a very individual dietary approach and no one meal fits all! In general, eating consistently every three (3) to five (5) hours and having three (3) nutritious well portioned meals a day together with two (2) healthful snacks can typically keep your blood sugar stable. However, according to individual needs (e.g., work schedule) some people find it useful to spread carbohydrates throughout the day to keep their blood sugar levels steady and others find it better to reduce the amount of carbohydrate in their diet to help control blood sugar levels without having an actual meal plan. A dietary assessment on the amount of carbohydrate in your food/drink and current meal pattern vis-à-vis your activity level is important to be discussed with a dietitian, so that right amount of carbohydrates is individually recommended.

Overall, foods containing carbohydrates can be replaced for each other in a meal plan. This does not mean that you can have a sugary food for dinner and a sweet for dessert! A meal plan with high quantities of added sugar will contribute to weight gain and a lower sense of fullness, which predisposes you to eat more. Therefore, a combination of fibre-rich carbohydrates with lean protein and heart-healthy fats (see section on Health Eating) are key to promote more stable glucose levels.

E) Reading the Food label
Food labels are an essential tool that provides further nutritional details on the product consumed and can therefore help you make better choices for meal planning and ultimately blood sugar control. For example, the ingredients are listed in descending order by weight, which means the ingredient with the highest amount in the product is listed first, followed by other ingredients used in decreasing order. This list can also show the level of food processing such as added salt or added sugars. Whole-grain products will contain more fibre which helps decrease sugar level spikes. It is not the purpose of this chapter to explain in detail food labels, but to simply to summarise the main issues of food labelling in relation to diabetes. A good summary on what is a nutrition claim and the ones

permitted can be found at 2022 European Commission Nutrition Claims.[8] For more practical information on food labels refer to the information provided by the Maltese Health Promotion and Disease Prevention Directorate (HPDPD) on the website shown in the reference list below.[9]

i.   Sugars-free products: A common misconception in diabetes is to look only at the quantity of sugars on the food label, denoted as 'of which sugars'. It is recommended to calculate the grams of total carbohydrates, including simple sugars, complex carbohydrates, and fibre, rather than the grams of simple sugars alone. If you emphasise on sugar content alone, you could miss out on healthy foods that contain natural sugar, such as milk and fruit. On the other hand, you might eat more foods with no natural or added sugars but have more processed carbohydrates, such as grains and cereals. These will still have an impact on blood sugar levels, especially if eaten in quantities more than your body needs. In relation to this notion, it is important that you do not just seek to buy 'Sugars-Free' products, as this does not mean that the food product is carbohydrate- free. When a choice is made between a standard product and their sugars-free equivalents, compare the food label; if the sugars-free product has less carbohydrates, then the sugar-free product could be a better choice. However, it also important to look at other ingredients to make a better healthy selection.

ii.   No-Added Sugars products: A claim of 'With No Added Sugars' or 'Contains Naturally Occurring Sugars' does not imply that the product does not have carbohydrates. Such products do not contain elevated sugar ingredients and will not have added sugar in the course of processing or packaging. Still, they may be high in carbohydrate load. Another common ingredient found on food

---

[8] European Commission (2022) Nutrition Claims. Available at: https://food.ec.europa.eu/safety/labelling-and-nutrition/nutrition-and-health-claims/nutrition- claims_en Accessed 1 November 2022.
[9] HPDPD (2011) Health Promotion and Disease Prevention Directorate. Available at: https://deputyprimeminister.gov.mt/en/health-promotion/Pages/Library/publications.aspx Accessed 15 October 2022.

labels are 'sugar alcohols' such as xylitol, sorbitol, and mannitol. Such products do not necessarily mean that they are low in carbohydrates or calories. Low carbohydrate food product may contain more calories, fats and/or proteins. So, it important that you look at the food ingredients before making them part of your meal planning.

iii.   Fat-Free products: The fat nutrient has more than double the calories of carbohydrates or proteins. 'Fat-Free' food products are easily available, but such product do not mean they do not contain carbohydrates. 'Fat-Free' foods can have more carbohydrates and contain almost as many calories as the original form of the same food. In addition, it is important to look that the types of fat listed on the label (see section 3) as this gives a good indication of healthier choice of fats such as monounsaturated and polyunsaturated fats.

Healthy eating for managing your weight and preventing chronic disease
Extra weight increases the risk of many other health conditions such as diabetes, also cardiovascular disease (heart disease), and some cancers amongst others. Excess weight is also linked to poorer mental wellbeing. Therefore, managing your excess weight and preventing obesity in the long term is a very important consideration to conserve your health and wellbeing in future years.

A) Causes of weight gain and obesity
It is important to be aware of the need to avoid or manage weight gain and what can cause your weight to increase. Weight gain happens when calorie (energy) intake is consistently higher than your calorie (energy) needs. There are many causes that can contribute and these include your specific genes, and your age and these factors cannot be changed. Other causes include a high calorie and nutritionally imbalanced diet, lack of sleep and low physical, high sedentary activity levels. Sedentary activities include sitting down for long periods of time watching TV or playing computer games, for example. Some of the conditions in the community within which we live, can also increase our risk of gaining weight. These could include the easiness to obtain unhealthy foods. The affordability of healthy

22

foods compared to more nutrient-dense fast foods could also be a problem. Examples of unhealthier foods and drinks include highly processed, calorie-rich foods such as salted snacks, confectionery items, biscuits, deep fried foods, and sugary drinks. Large portion sizes can also contribute to faster weight gain.

B) Food-based dietary guidelines as a healthy eating guide
The plate model indicated in the figure below shows the six main food groups with the size of the segment matching the relative contribution for each food group in our daily diet:

- cereals and cereal products, especially wholegrain, and potatoes;
- lean meats, fish, poultry, eggs, legumes, unsalted nuts and seeds;
- fruits;
- vegetables;
- milk and milk products;
- fats and oils.

A 'Mediterranean diet' eating style is recommended rather than a typical 'Westernized' diet which is usually higher in processed foods, saturated fats and refined carbohydrates. Following a Mediterranean diet means making the shift towards reducing red and processed meat intake, to eating more plant-based foods such as legumes, fruit, and vegetables, including vegetable oils (such as olive oil) instead of animal foods high in saturated fats such as butter, cheeses, and creams. There is evidence today that a Mediterranean diet reduces the risk of chronic disease including diabetes amongst other health benefits.[10,11]

---

[10] Huo, R. et al. (2014) "Effects of mediterranean-style diet on glycemic control, weight loss and cardiovascular risk factors among type 2 diabetes individuals: A meta-analysis," European Journal of Clinical Nutrition, 69(11), pp. 1200–1208. Available at: https://doi.org/10.1038/ejcn.2014.243.
[11] Esposito, K. et al. (2015) "A Journey into a Mediterranean diet and type 2 diabetes: A systematic review with Meta-analyses," BMJ Open, 5(8). Available at: https://doi.org/10.1136/bmjopen-2015-008222.

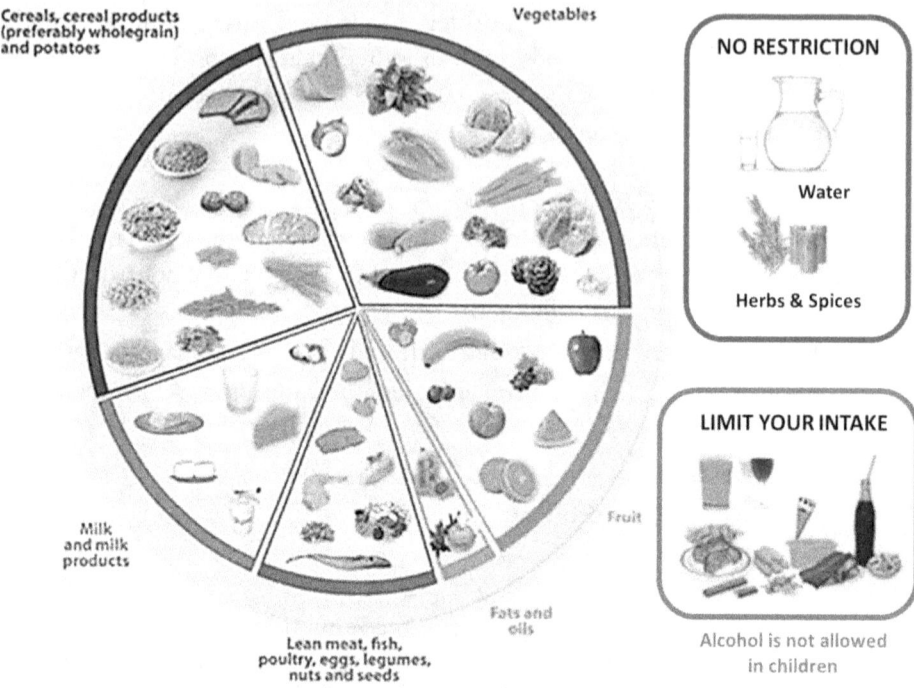

Cereals, cereal products (preferably wholegrain) and potatoes

Vegetables

NO RESTRICTION

Water

Herbs & Spices

LIMIT YOUR INTAKE

Alcohol is not allowed in children

Milk and milk products

Fruit

Fats and oils

Lean meat, fish, poultry, eggs, legumes, nuts and seeds

The Health Plate – A Mediterranean diet guide for eating throughout life [12]
Select a variety of nutritious foods from each food group every day. Drink plenty of water. Keep active. Reduce sitting time. Enjoy your meals with family and friends.

C) Weight loss in a safe and sustainable way

A simple measure for checking your weight according to your height is by calculating your Body Mass Index (BMI). The BMI consists of measuring your height (in metres) and weight (in kilograms) and then carrying out the calculation below:

$$\frac{\text{Weight(kg)}}{[\text{height(m)}]^2}$$

---

[12] Modified from: Ministry of Health, Elderly and Care (2016) Dietary Guidelines for Maltese adults. Available at: healthy plate en.pdf (gov.mt). Accessed 5 November 2022

If your BMI is over 25 kg/m2 and lower than 29.9 kg/m2 then it falls in the overweight category, a BMI over 30 kg/m2 falls within the obesity range. Ideally, you should always aim to keep your BMI within the range of 18.5-24.9 kg/m2. If you need to lose some weight, then the weight loss should be slow and sustainable. Aim for approximately 0.5-1.0 kg/weekly weight loss rate when possible. Remember that even small to modest reductions in weight (5-10% of your weight) can contribute to health gains such as reducing the risk of diabetes.[13] Indeed, it was proposed that weight loss of 5 to15% should be a key target of management for persons living with type 2 diabetes.[14]

D) Eating tips for safe and sustainable weight loss
- Make small changes to your current typical eating patterns, for example, by drinking water instead of sugary drinks
- Keep track of your daily meals and monitor your progress
- Watch out for your portion sizes, these should reflect your overall calorie needs for weight loss
- Eat small meals spaced throughout the day
- Increase your physical activity habits for example, take the stairs instead of the lift or walk to your appointments rather than use transport
- Reduce your sedentary behaviours and plan little activity breaks during long sitting periods
- Reduce your alcohol intake, remember that alcohol contains a substantial amount of calories which will work against your weight loss targets apart from causing other undesirable effects
- Set targets that are practical and reachable for you to keep
- Maintain your weight once you achieve your targets by keeping to a healthy balanced diet

[13] Jensen, M.D. et al. (2014) "2013 AHA/ACC/TOS guideline for the management of overweight and obesity in adults," Journal of the American College of Cardiology, 63(25), pp. 2985–3023. Available at: https://doi.org/10.1016/j.jacc.2013.11.004.
[14] Lingvay, I. et al. (2022) "Obesity management as a primary treatment goal for type 2 diabetes: Time to reframe the conversation," The Lancet, 399(10322), pp. 394–405. Available at: https://doi.org/10.1016/s0140-6736(21)01919-x.

Conclusion

Dietary control and managing your weight are key to diabetes management and prevention. This must be done with the primary aim of encouraging and supporting sustainable patterns of healthy eating, focusing on the nutrition requirements of the individual, keeping the pleasure of eating, and offering the necessary tools for improving healthy eating.[15] There is no particular percentage of carbohydrate, proteins and fat intake that is ideal for all persons with diabetes. There is no diabetes diet or 'one diet-fits-all'. Instead, individually designated meal plans that highlight foods with demonstrated health benefits that accommodate individual preferences in a practical way is key for blood sugar control. Such recommendations are useless without individuals with diabetes participating in their own care. As a matter of fact, research has shown that if you participate in your own care, there is a greater impact on the prevention, development, and progression of diabetes.[16]

Average total carbohydrate content of commonly consumed foods

Food Item	Typical Portion Size	Carbohydrate per portion (g)
BREADS		
Burger roll	1 larger (82g)	40
Ciabatta roll	1 average roll (97g)	50
Croissant	1 average (50g)	20
Crusty white roll	1 average (50g)	30
Granary bread	1 medium slice (36g)	15
Muffin	1 average (68g)	25
Pitta Bread	1 medium (69g)	38
White Bread	1 medium slice (33g)	15
Wholemeal bread	1 medium slice (36g)	15

---

[15] Davies, M.J. et al. (2022) "Management of hyperglycemia in type 2 diabetes, 2022. A consensus report by the American Diabetes Association (ADA) and the European Association for the Study of Diabetes (EASD)," Diabetes Care, 45(11), pp. 2753–2786. Available at: https://doi.org/10.2337/dci22-0034

[16] Shrivastava, S.R.B.L., Shrivastava, P.S. and Ramasamy, J. (2013) "Role of self-care in management of diabetes mellitus," Journal of Diabetes & Metabolic Disorders, 12(1). Available at: https://doi.org/10.1186/2251-6581-12-14.

RICE/PASTA

Couscous (raw)	1 tablespoon (12g)	9
Egg Noodles (dry)	1 dry sheet / nest (63g)	45
White pasta such as macaroni, fusilli, penne dried, uncooked	75g	53
Spaghetti (uncooked)	75g	53
Ravioli	1 average ready meal (250g)	66
Rice (uncooked)	1 tablespoon (18g)	14
Tortellini (cooked)	180g	47

BREAKFAST CEREALS

All Bran	6 tablespoons (40g)	20
Bran Flakes	5 tablespoons (40g)	30
Cornflakes	6 tablespoons (30g)	25
Fruit and nut muesli	4 tablespoons (50g)	35
Fruit'n Fibre	6 tablespoons (35g)	25
Porridge	27g sachet + 180ml milk	25
Special K	7 tablespoons (30g)	22.5
Weetabix	1 biscuit (20g)	13

BISCUITS

Cereal Bar	1 average	15
Digestive	1 biscuit	10
Plain crackers	2 cream crackers (16g)	10

BUNS & CAKES

Almond slice	1 average slice (33g)	20
Carrot cake (iced)	1 average slice (60g)	32
Doughnut (jam)	1 average (71g)	49
Doughnut (ring)	1 average (66g)	47
Fruit cake	plain 1 small (60g)	36
Hot cross bun	1 average (51g)	30
Jam tart	1 small (34g)	23
Mince pie	1 average (60g)	36
Strawberry/black forest gateau	1 slice (135g)	50
Apple pie	Average slice (100g)	36

DAIRY/DESSERTS		
Dried skimmed milk powder	1 teaspoon	3
Fresh milk (all types)	200ml (1/3 pint)	10
Diet (Light) yoghurt	Small pot (125g)	10
Yoghurt	Small pot (125g)	22
Custard (made-up)	200ml	32
FRUIT		
Apple	Medium (150g)	18
Apricots dried	4 ready to eat (40g)	15
Banana (no skin)	1 medium (85g)	20
Grapefruit	Half (120g)	5
Grapes	10 average (65g)	10
Kiwi fruit	1 average (50g)	5
Melon eg Honeydew	1 slice (100g)	7
Nectarine	1 medium (140g)	12
Orange (with skin)	1 medium (115g)	7
Peach	1 medium (125g)	9
Pear	1 medium (200g)	20
Pineapple	fresh 1 ring (40g)	4
Plum	2 average (110g)	10
Prunes (dried)	2 medium (30g)	10
Raisins	1 tablespoon (30g)	20
Strawberries	7 average	5
VEGETABLES		
Potatoes (uncooked)	1 medium (60g)	10
Sweetcorn (canned)	2tbsp (67g)	18
Peas (boiled)	2tbsp (60g)	6
Kidney beans (cooked/canned)	2tbsp (65g)	12
Chickpeas (cooked/canned)	2tbsp (70g)	11
Baked beans	2tbsp (120g)	18
Carrots (raw)	100g	10
Onions (raw)	100g	9

Self-monitoring of Blood Glucose [1]

Introduction

Why is self monitoring necessary? Glucose monitoring performed by persons with diabetes and by the health care team attending these individuals is an integral feature of diabetes care to ensure that short and long-term complications are avoided. Persons with diabetes can manage their condition effectively and safely only if they are able to perform self-monitoring of blood glucose on a regular basis.

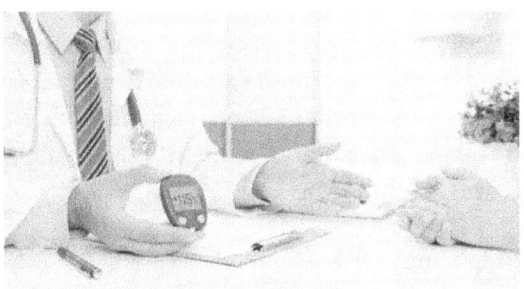

Monitoring should be performed regularly and accurately. This facilitates better glycaemic control and significantly reduces the risk of onset or delay the progression of complications. However, it is essential that to be able to understand the significance of the results obtained and the actions that need to be taken, the person with diabetes has to be aware of:

o The individual set targets of treatment.
o The signs, symptoms and problems of diabetes.
o How to cope with hyperglycaemia and acute illness.
o Food interactions with physical activity and the diabetic treatment.
o The individual nutritional requirements and meal planning.
o Factors promoting improvement in lifestyle.
o The adverse effects of smoking and alcohol.

---

[1] Prepared by Ms. Moira Grixti.

Significance of self-monitoring of blood glucose

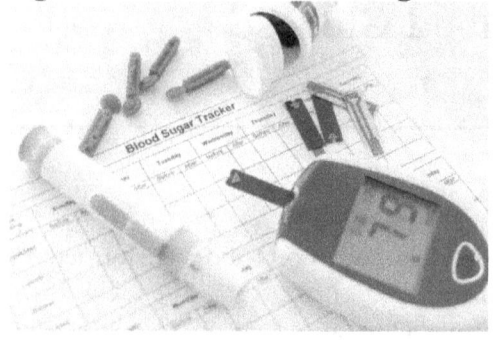 Self-monitoring is a means of achieving a goal rather than a goal in itself. It is of great importance for the individual to always keep an accurate record of the results. When completing the Monitoring Diary, it is important also to record the hypoglycaemic and any other treatment you may have been prescribed in the long or short-term, and the time of day you are meant to be taking the treatment. Very often, your doctor or diabetes nurse may indicate the ideal time during the day to perform blood glucose monitoring.

Blood glucose monitoring is an important tool in the management of diabetes and the prevention of complications. Persons living with diabetes need to ensure that whenever they have a visit either in hospital or at their GP or diabetes nurse, they should always have their blood glucose monitoring diary with them.

It is important to take note that:
o   Severe dehydration and excessive water loss may cause readings which are higher than the actual values.
o   If the blood glucose results are lower or higher than usual, and one does not have any symptoms of being unwell, repeat the test.

It is important to increase the monitor frequency if:
o   The hypoglycaemic treatment has been adjusted or changed.
o   If there are any sign or symptoms of hypoglycaemia (low blood glucose of less than 3.9 mmol/l).
o   Physical activity has increased.
o   You feel unwell.
o   You have to fast for a period of time [say before surgery].
o   In preparation of embarking on a pregnancy or during pregnancy.

Regular self-monitoring of blood glucose is advantageous, because:
- It is critical to quantify the safety of treatment. and
- It is necessary for good management of diabetes.
- It reduce the risk of overdosage with subsequent hypoglycaemic attacks.
- It can prevent hyperglycaemia and ketoacidosis.
- It can help to adjust diet.
- It can help to adjust the treatment to exercise levels.
- It prevents long-term complications.
- It can help decrease the mortality rate from complication of diabetes.
- It improves quality of life by empowering the person with diabetes providing the tools to manage ones own health.

Self-monitoring testing procedure

The procedure to carry out glucose self-monitoring involves obtaining a drop of blood, generally from the fingertip. Precautions must be taken at all times to reduce the risks of getting an infection at the puncture site.

Before puncturing the fingertip:
- Never share a lancet or the lancing device with anybody else.
- Always use a new, sterile lancet. Lancets are for single use only.
- Avoid getting hand lotion oils, dirt, or debris in or on the lancets and the lancing device.
- Wash your hands with soap and water.
- Dry your hands.
- Select the puncture site at fingertips. Choose a different spot each time you test. Repeated punctures at the same spot may cause soreness and calluses.
- Rub the puncture site for about 20 seconds before pricking your finger.
- Press the lancing device's tip firmly against the lower side of your fingertip. Press the release button to prick your finger, then a click indicates that the puncture is complete.
- It is recommended that you discard the first drop of blood as it might contain tissue fluid, which may affect the test result.

Furthermore, to ensure the accuracy and reliability of the blood glucose meter quality control checks having quality control solutions should be carried out. Quality control solutions should always be available to be purchased at the supplier /pharmacy.

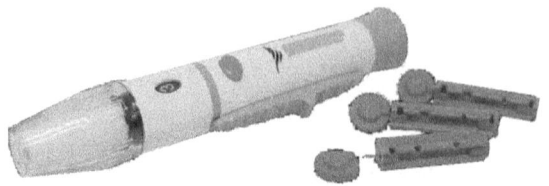

Lancets and Lancing device

Performing the Blood Glucose Test:
- Insert the test strip to turn on the meter.
- Obtaining a blood sample: Use the pre-set lancing device to puncture the desired site. Wipe off the first appeared drop of blood with a clean cotton swab. Gently squeeze the punctured area to obtain another drop of blood. Be careful NOT to smear the blood sample.
- Apply the blood drop onto the test strip.
- Read your result: The result of your blood glucose test will appear after the meter counts down to 0. The blood glucose result will be stored in the memory automatically.
- Eject the test strip by pushing the eject button on the side. Use a sharp bin to dispose of used test strips. The meter will switch itself off automatically.

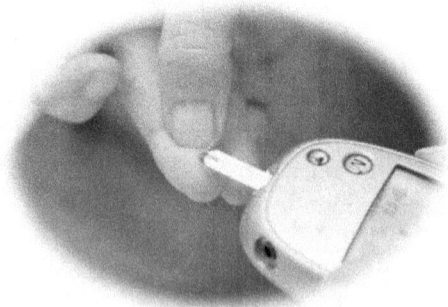

Testing fingertip blood using a glucose meter

Blood glucose monitoring timing

The ideal frequency and timing of checking one's blood glucose should be discussed with the doctor or diabetes nurse. This will often depend on the severity of the diabetes and the treatment one is taking to control the condition. Blood glucose self-monitoring is generally carried out:

o   Before breakfast and 2 hours after breakfast
o   Before Lunch and 2 hours after lunch
o   Before Dinner and 2hours after dinner
o   And at Bedtime

Blood Glucose Monitoring should be done before taking any treatment whether this involves the administration of insulin and/or oral diabetes medication. During pregnancy, testing should be carried out before a meal and 1 hour after the meal and again at bedtime.

Recommended blood glucose targets

Ideal blood glucose targets are individualized and dependent upon:

o   Duration of Diabetes
o   Age/life expectancy
o   Co-morbidities
o   Cardiovascular disease or diabetes complications
o   Hypoglycaemia unawareness
o   Individual patient consideration

The table below shows ideal blood glucose levels before and after meals for people with and without diabetes.

	Non-diabetics	Diabetic persons
Fasting	70-99 mg/dl 3.9-5.5 mmol/L	80-130 mg/dl 4.4-7.2 mmol/L
1-2 hours after meals	<140 mg/dl <7.8 mmol/L	<180 mg/dl <7.0 mmol/L

What is continuous glucose monitoring?

Self-monitoring blood glucose using a blood glucose meter provides only a single measurement at the time of the test. This may be done several times a day, however the accuracy of the glycaemic picture obtained is limited and not necessarily totally accurate. To obtain a near accurate picture of the glycaemic state of the person with diabetes, one would need to perform multiple blood glucose testing which is difficult and inconvenient to perform.

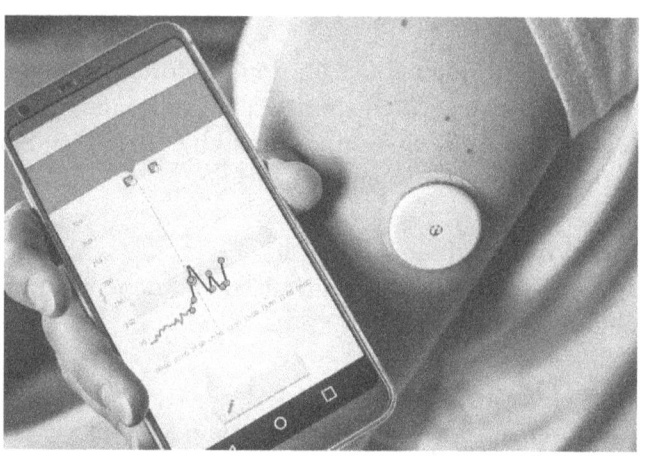

Continuous glucose monitoring (CGM) is one of the most important recent advances in diabetes technology to provide better diabetes management. CGM automatically tracks blood glucose levels throughout the day and night providing an accurate picture of the daily glycaemic state of the person. It also easily allows the person living with diabetes to see the glucose level anytime. Thus, one can review how the blood glucose levels change over a few hours or days allowing the person to see overall glucose level trends. Seeing glucose levels in real-time can assist a person living with diabetes make more informed decisions in making lifestyle modifications in order to effectively manage the diabetes by decreasing the time spent in low and high blood glucose ranges. A vast number of studies have confirmed that CGM can improve blood glucose control which in turn reduce the complications associated with diabetes.

How does a continuous glucose monitor (CGM) work?

A CGM works by placing a tiny sensor inserted under the skin, usually in the arm or abdomen. Depending on the model available, the sensor will need to be replaced every 10 or 14 days. The sensor measures the glucose levels in the fluid between the cells [interstitial glucose levels] every few minutes. A wireless transmitter sends the information to a monitor or directly to a smartphone. CGM is the ideal self-monitoring tool for persons with Type 1 Diabetes whose glycaemic status is very fragile and likely to fluctuate markedly. CGM is highly recommended for those who:

o Are on Intensive insulin therapy, also called tight blood glucose control, requiring to test blood glucose more than 8 times a day.

o Experience severe hypoglycaemia and have hypoglycaemia unawareness, i.e., do not sense the symptoms that their blood glucose is going low (below 4mmol/l).

o Type 1 diabetic women who are pregnant or are planning a pregnancy.

o Those who practice intense physical or sports activities.

Glucose levels are recorded continuously at all times of the day and night, whether one is showering, working, at school, exercising, or sleeping.

Modern CGMs have added features acting on the glucose readings. Thus:

o The CGM may have an alarm incorporated to react to too low or too high glucose levels alerting the person with diabetes to take immediate action. Of course, because CGMs test interstitial glucose levels, and these may not truly reflect the real-time blood glucose levels, it is very important that before taking any remedial action in response to the alarm, the glucose values need to be confirmed by using a blood glucose meter before making any treatment decisions.

o One can input the timing of meals, physical activity, doses of insulin taken alongside the glucose levels allowing the person to visualize the real-time effects of exercise, meals, or treatment on glucose levels.

o Data can be downloaded onto a computer or smart device to easily plot glucose level trends. These results can be used to adjust insulin doses and provide insight as to the potential cause for glucose excursions.

o   Some models can send information right away to a second person's smartphone—perhaps a parent, partner, or healthcare provider. For example, if the glucose drops dangerously low overnight, the CGM could be set to alert the parent/partner/caregiver wherever they may be, to assist accordingly.

CGM therefore significantly empowers the person living with diabetes and definitely improves their quality of life. While healthcare costs are likely to increase if CGM is made available for all persons living with Type 1 diabetes, the long-term health care costs will however definitely be reduced as a result of better blood glucose control which will help reduce the risks for complications leading to decreasing unnecessary hospital admissions.

Pharmacological management of diabetes [1]

Introduction

Type 1 and type 2 diabetes are complex diseases commonly occurring in the setting of hypertension and high lipid levels [dyslipidaemia]). Unfortunately, both increase the risk of potentially fatal and/or disabling complications affecting the large arteries (coronary artery disease leading to heart attacks, cerebrovascular disease leading to strokes, disease of the peripheral circulation leading to limb loss/amputations) and small arteries (retinopathy [disease of the retina in the eye], nephropathy [kidney disease] and neuropathy [disease of the nervous system]). The complications can be avoided by adequate pharmacological medication to help maintain normal blood glucose levels.

Type 1 diabetes, characterised by irreversible destruction of the pancreatic beta cells by autoantibodies, necessitates lifelong lifesaving insulin therapy. On the other hand, the pathological hallmark of type 2 diabetes, namely resistance to the effects of insulin (insulin resistance) permits the use of several oral and injectable insulin-sparing glucose lowering agents, even as beta-cell failure sets in. Treatment with insulin sparing agents in type 2 diabetes is generally considered less burdensome, although most of such patients will require insulin therapy at a later stage of their disease. This review aims explain the salient characteristics and rationale behind the use of different pharmacological agents in the management of type 1 and type 2 diabetes.

---

[1] Prepared by Dr. Sando Vella.

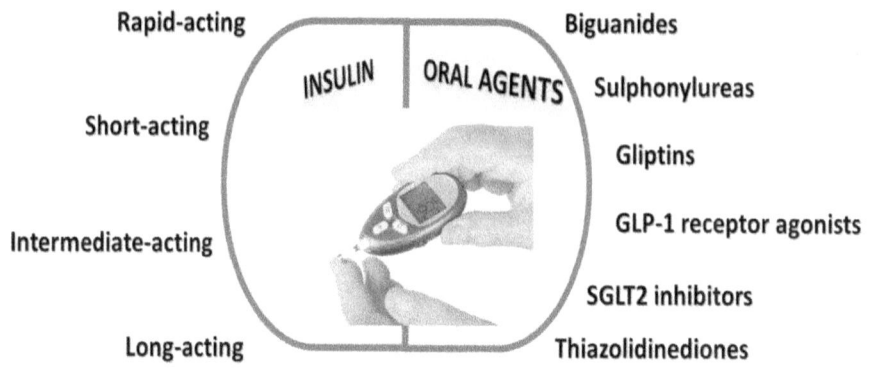

Rapid-acting		Biguanides
Short-acting	INSULIN | ORAL AGENTS	Sulphonylureas
		Gliptins
Intermediate-acting		GLP-1 receptor agonists
		SGLT2 inhibitors
Long-acting		Thiazolidinediones

Hypoglycaemic agents

Biguanides – Metformin

Metformin is currently advocated as initial glucose lowering therapy in type 2 diabetes, typically achieving an HbA1c reduction of 0.8 to 1.0% (9-12 mmol/mol). Derived from the French Lilac plant *Galega officinalis*, it acts as a weak insulin sensitizer which lowers blood glucose levels by (i) reducing the generation of glucose through breakdown of glucagon in the liver (gluconeogenesis) and (ii) promoting insulin mediating glucose uptake and metabolism by skeletal muscle.

The main advantages of metformin can be summarised as follows:

- It is cheap and effective - hence its position as first line agent in the pharmacological management of type 2 diabetes. This is particularly relevant is lower income countries, particularly if patients need to fund their own treatment.
- Weight neutral – use of metformin is not associated with significant weight increase or loss.
- Potential benefits on cardiovascular outcomes. The landmark UK Prospective Diabetes Study (UKPDS) had reported (albeit in a small number of patients) that use of metformin was associated with a reduced risk of myocardial infarction (heart attacks) and all-cause mortality.

Potential adverse effects of metformin therapy include the following:

- Gastrointestinal – nausea, bloating, diarrhoea, abdominal pains. This is an unpredictable side effect which can be minimised by introducing at a lowest dose (500 mg daily) and increasing the total daily dose gradually. Use of sustained release metformin preparations are also associated with a lower risk of gastrointestinal adverse effects.

- Lactic acidosis – accumulation of lactic acid in body tissues is a serious adverse effect, development of which is however highly unlikely provided metformin is used in the correct clinical setting. To this end, metformin should be prescribed with caution in type 2 diabetes patients with moderate renal and liver impairment. Its use is contraindicated in patients with end stage kidney and liver disease. Moreover, metformin should not be prescribed in the setting of acute severe illness (such as severe infections) causing a significant drop in blood pressure, severe dehydration, and recurrent vomiting.

- Vitamin B12 deficiency – metformin reduces intestinal absorption of vitamin B12 in up to 30% of patients and lowers serum vitamin B12 levels in up to 5-10% of patients who have been treated with metformin for five years. Periodic testing of vitamin B12 levels should be considered in patients treated with metformin, especially in the setting of peripheral neuropathy or anaemia, of in patients particularly at risk of vitamin B12 deficiency such as vegans or patients who have undergone bariatric surgery.

Sulphonylureas

Sulphonylureas are cheap rapidly effective glucose lowering agents that act by stimulating the beta cells of the islets of pancreas to secrete insulin through their binding to a specific channel at the surface of the aforementioned cells. They include gliclazide, glimepiride and glipizide, as well as the older generation (and longer acting) glibenclamide. Sulphonylurea use is associated with an HbA1c reduction of 0.8 – 2.0% (9-22 mmol/mol).

In contrast to metformin and newer generation oral glucose lowering agents, sulphonylurea use has not been associated with drug-specific improvement in cardiovascular outcomes. Traditionally prescribed as 'second line agents' in the management of type 2 diabetes (after metformin), their role is largely being replaced by newer and safer oral glucose lowering agents, particularly those with proven benefits on cardiovascular and kidney-related outcomes.

The major adverse effects of sulphonylureas are:

- Weight gain – this occurs by virtue of the mechanism of action of this class of drugs. A landmark type 2 diabetes trial called the United Kingdom Prospective Diabetes Study (UKPDS) reported a mean weight gain of 2.5 kg after 10 years of therapy.
- Hypoglycaemia – this is a major adverse effect and is particularly worrisome for the longer acting sulphonylurea glibenclamide. At least half of type 2 diabetes patients treated with a sulphonylurea may experience at least one hypoglycaemic episode per year. The risk of sustaining such an adverse event increase in patients with significant kidney and liver disease.

Caution should be exercised when prescribing such drugs to elderly and frail patients. Sulhonylureas should not be prescribed in patients with porphyria.

Gliptins – Dipeptidyl peptidase IV inhibitors

Like GLP-1 receptor agonists (discussed below), dipeptidyl peptidase IV (DPP-IV) inhibitors act on the incretin system. The incretin hormone GLP-1 is secreted by the L cells of the distal ileum and colon in response to a meal and stimulates insulin secretion by the beta cells of the islets of pancreas. However, GLP-1 has a very short duration of action (half-life = 2 minutes), it being broken down by an enzyme called dipeptidyl peptidase IV (DPP-IV). Several of these agents have been introduced in the market in recent years, including sitagliptin, vildagliptin, linagliptin, saxagliptin and alogliptin. Their use typically causes an HbA1c reduction of 0.4% (5 mmol/mol).

The main advantages of gliptins can be summarised as follows:

- weight neutral
- low risk of hypoglycaemia
- their cardiovascular safety has been well documented in large well-designed cardiovascular outcome studies. However, their use has not been associated with drug-specific cardiovascular benefits.

40

Concerns have been reported regarding a possible association of saxagliptin (and possibly alogliptin) with an increased risk of hospitalization for heart failure. This observation has not been observed among patients treated with sitagliptin. Sitagliptin, saxagliptin, vildagliptin and alogliptin requires dose reduction in the setting of significant kidney disease; linagliptin can be continued in these circumstances. Use of DPP-IV inhibitors has been associated with an increased risk of pancreatitis and bullous pemphigoid. To this end, this class of drugs should not be prescribed in patients with a past history of pancreatitis.

GLP-1 receptor agonists

In addition to promoting glucose-dependent insulin secretion, these injectable agents inhibit the secretion of glucagon (which antagonises insulin secretion), slows down stomach emptying (at least in the short term) and suppresses interest in food through its action on an appetite-regulating (satiety) centre located in a part of the brain called the hypothalamus. Initial agents- such as exenatide require once daily (liraglutide, lixisenatide) or twice daily (exenatide) administration. Later, novel extended release GLP-1 receptor agonists were introduced, permitting once weekly administration (exenatide extended release, semaglutide, and dulaglutide). Subcutaneous administration of these drugs occurs using a pen injecting device, delivering the relevant GLP-1 analogue into fat beneath the skin, much akin to insulin therapy administration. GLP-1 receptor agonists achieve an HbA1c reduction of 0.5 – 1.8% (6-20 mmol/mol). Shorter acting GLP-1 receptor agonists tend to have a greater effect on glucose excursions after meals and stomach emptying, while longer acting agents are more likely to affect fasting glucose levels, with a weaker efficacy on glucose elevations after meals. Semaglutide has recently been introduced as an oral agent.

The major advantages of GLP-1 receptor agonists can be summarised as follows:

- Weight loss – of up to 6kg has been noted in patients prescribed GLP-1 receptor agonists. This favourable effect is most pronounced among patients prescribed semaglutide, followed (in decreasing order) by liraglutide, dulaglutide, exenatide and lixisenatide.

- Low risk of hypoglycaemia – by virtue of their mechanism of action, use of GLP-1 receptor agonists carries a very low risk of hypoglycaemia in clinical settings. This adverse effect is more likely to happen if a particular GLP-1 analogue is prescribed with other glucose lowering agents such as sulphonylureas or insulin. In this setting, addition of GLP-1 receptor agonists may necessitate a reduction in the prevailing dose of co-prescribed drug and closer monitoring of glucose readings.

- Improved cardiovascular outcomes – available evidence arising out of well-designed cardiovascular outcome trials for liraglutide, dulaglutide and semaglutide (once weekly) demonstrated that GLP-1 receptor agonists lower the risk of major cardiovascular events in patients with established or at high risk of cardiovascular disease. In a systematic review and meta-analysis, once weekly exetanide, liraglutide and semaglutide also reduced cardiovascular mortality in type 2 diabetes patients with established cardiovascular disease. Use of GLP-1 receptor agonists has also been linked to a reduction in prevailing cholesterol levels and blood pressure readings. The precise mechanism underpinning the latter benefits remains elusive, perhaps a consequence of drug-associated weight loss. Unlike SGLT2 inhibitors (discussed below), GLP-1 receptor agonists have no effect on heart failure rates or outcomes.

- Improved renal outcomes – Current evidence suggests a role for liraglutide, semaglutide and dulaglutide in reducing adverse kidney related outcomes in type 2 diabetes patients. However, the extent and mechanism of this beneficial effect needs to be clarified by specifically designed clinical studies.

In terms of adverse effects, prescription of GLP-1 receptor agonists has been associated with early satiety, nausea, vomiting and diarrhoea, affecting up to 50% of treated patients. However, such complications are usually transient. Despite initial concerns regarding a possible association of GLP-1 receptor agonists with pancreatitis and pancreatic cancer, data from observational and randomised controlled trials have not confirmed any possible cause and effect relationship. Nonetheless, given these concerns, GLP-1 receptor agonists are not recommended in patients with a history of pancreatitis. Semaglutide has been associated with an increased risk of retinopathy and its complications. However, this is more likely in patients with background retinopathy, and in whom, glycaemic control rapidly improved following initiation of therapy. Given observations of higher benign and malignant medullary thyroid tumours in rodent studies (albeit not in humans), GLP-1 analogues should not be prescribed in patients with a personal or family history of medullary thyroid carcinoma or deemed at increased genetic risk of such tumours (MEN 2A or 2B).

Use of GLP-1 receptor agonists is additionally contraindicated in patients with type 1 diabetes, type 2 diabetes patients known to suffer from delayed stomach emptying (gastroparesis- typically in patients with autonomic neuropathy), and significantly impaired renal function (EGFR < 30 mls/min/1.73 m2 for exenatide twice daily and lixisenatide; EGFR < 45 for exenatide once weekly formulation). Liraglutide, semaglutide and dulaglutide may be continued as standard doses even in patients with an estimated glomerular filtration rate < 30 mls/min/1.73 m2

SGLT2 inhibitors

SGLT2 inhibitors constitute another novel class of oral glucose lowering agents which enhance the excretion of glucose in the urine. This is achieved through blocking the reabsorption of glucose by as much as 90% in a section of the filtering mechanism of the kidney called the proximal renal tubule. Given their mechanism, their glucose lowering effect is greatest in patients with relatively preserved and intact kidney function. SGLT2 inhibitors achieve an HbA1c improvement of 0.5 to 1.8% (6-20 mmol/mol).

Advantages
- Low risk of hypoglycaemia – as is the case for GLP-1 receptor agonists, use of SGLT-2 inhibitors is associated with a low risk of hypoglycaemia when prescribed alone or in combination with metformin. Risk increases when SGLT-2 inhibitors are added with sulphonylurea or insulin therapy – a reduction in the dose of the latter may be warranted, depending on prevailing glycaemic control.
- Weight loss – SGLT2 inhibitors are attractive as adjunct 2nd or 3rd line agents in patients in whom weight gain is particularly not desirable and GLP-1 receptor agonists are contraindicated or not desired. Weight loss is seemingly sustained, and approximates 3kg after 2 years of therapy.
- Blood pressure reduction – this is a modest drug-related effect.
- Improved cardiovascular outcomes – SGLT2 inhibitors have been shown in large cardiovascular outcome trials to reduce the risk of

cardiovascular events (canagliflozin, empagliflozin and dapagliflozin) and hospitalisation for heart failure (canagliflozin, empagliflozin, ertugliflozin, dapagliflozin) in patients with established or at high risk of cardiovascular disease. To this end, major diabetes guidelines advocate use of one of these agents in patients with a history of coronary artery disease or heart failure with reduced ejection fraction. To date, it remains unclear whether prescribing SGLT2 inhibitors to type 2 diabetes patients without established cardiovascular disease translates into beneficial effects on cardiovascular outcomes in the longer term.

- Improved renal outcomes – Canagliflozin, empagliflozin and dapagliflozin have been shown to afford renal protection in patients with an estimated glomerular filtration rate < 90 mls/min/1.73 m2. Overall benefit decreases in patients with significantly impaired renal function.

Adverse effects

- Urinary tract infections and genital trush – Use of SGLT2 inhibitors has been associated with an increased risk of balanitis in men, vaginitis in women and urinary tract infections. This is likely to occur as a direct consequence of the mechanism of action of these drugs – which as outlined above, promote the excretion of glucose in the urine, and hence the exposure of the genitourinary tract to high glucose levels. Recurrent urinary tract and genital infections necessitate SGLT2 inhibitor withdrawal or avoidance. Necrotizing fasciitis of the perineum is another rare adverse effect.

- Fractures – Some, but not all studies have reported an increased risk of fractures in patients treated with canagliflozin, possibly as a result of orthostatic hypotension and falls (see above). Canagliflozin has also been associated with worsening bone density at the hip and spine. Whether this observation holds true for other SGLT2 inhibitors remains to be established.

- Dehydration and orthostatic hypotension – by promoting glucose and water loss via the urinary tract. Caution should be exercised in the elderly, and in patients treated with angiontensin converting enzyme inhibitors, angiontensin II receptor blockers and diuretics.

- Euglycaemic diabetic ketoacidosis – this can be a diagnostic challenge, since the potentially deadly (if untreated) accumulation of ketoacids occurs in the absence of significantly high glucose levels. A high index of suspicion is warranted, and patients should be warned to stop their use of this drug in the setting of identifiable precipitating scenarios, such as severe infection (sepsis) and dehydration. Risk of diabetic ketoacidosis is highest with canagliflozin therapy.

- Amputations – Canagliflozin therapy has been associated with an increased risk of lower limb amputations (predominantly midfoot and toe). Patients known to suffer from peripheral arterial disease, neuropathy or a previous history of amputation are at highest risk of such an adverse effect – prescription of SGLT2 inhibitors is best avoided in this setting. Indeed, risk of this adverse effect with canagliflozin has been mitigated in later trials by meticulous and regular foot examinations, and SGLT2 inhibitor withdrawal in patients deemed at higher risk of this adverse effect. To date, the association of other SGLT2 inhibitors with an increased risk of amputations remains unclear, with different studies reporting conflicting outcomes.

SGLT2 inhibitors are contraindicated in patients with type 1 diabetes, a history of diabetic ketoacidosis and should be used with caution in patients with a history of amputation (or risk factors for amputation – as outlined above) or deemed at higher risk of diabetic ketoacidosis (pancreatic insufficiency, history of ethanol or drug abuse, ketogenic diets).

Thiazolidinediones

Thiazolidinediones are insulin sensitizing agents that activate the PPAR-γ receptor. Troglitazone and later rosiglitazone were withdrawn from the market on account of worrisome adverse effects (fatal liver failure and increased cardiovascular mortality respectively). Pioglitazone remains the only available drug in this class, classically resulting in an HbA1c reduction of 0.6 -1.5% (7-17 mmmol/mol).

Unfortunately, widespread use of pioglitazone has been hampered by its association with weight gain, fluid retention and heart failure. To this end, pioglitazone should not be prescribed in patients with a history of heart failure. Its use should also be avoided in patients with a history of bladder cancer and in patients who suffer from or are deemed at an increased risk of osteoporosis, given a reported association with bone fractures. Nonetheless, use of pioglitazone has been reported to reduce the risk of cardiovascular events among patients with established or deemed at risk of cardiovascular disease.

Less commonly used oral glucose lowering agents include α-glucosidase inhibitors (such as acarbose) and prandial insulin secretagogues (such as repaglinide and nateglinide). α glucosidase inhibitors antagonise the breakdown of carbohydrates into monosaccharides (simple sugars) within the digestive tract, effectively lowering glucose peaks after meals. However, passage of undigested carbohydrates into the large intestine increases the risk bloating and diarrhoea. Repaglinide and nateglinide stimulate insulin secretion but have a much shorter duration of action than the more widely prescribed sulphonylureas, hence lowering risk of hypoglycaemia.

Insulins

Despite the ever-increasing range of non-insulin glucose lowering agents, insulin remains pivotal in the management of type 2 diabetes, particularly in patients with long duration of the disease, when beta cell failure had reached such an advanced stage that other glucose lowering options do not suffice in controlling prevailing blood glucose levels. Insulin is indispensable and lifesaving treatment for patients with type 1 diabetes, in whom beta-cell destruction by antibodies precludes the secretion of this essential hormone. A variety of insulin preparations and insulin dosing strategies are available – choice is dictated by patient and doctor preference, glycaemic control, and lifestyle factors.

Insulin is a drug with a narrow therapeutic window: too much insulin will inevitably lead to hypoglycaemia while too little insulin will fail to achieve adequate glycaemic control. Hence, the decision to proceed with insulin therapy needs to be accompanied by adequate patient training and support and a commitment regarding frequent glucose monitoring. Information derived from self-monitoring of blood glucose aids the caring clinician to achieve safe glucose targets by titrating the patient's insulin dose as required.

Over the years, multiple and different insulin preparations, each with its characteristic peak time and duration of action, have become available for use by clinicians.

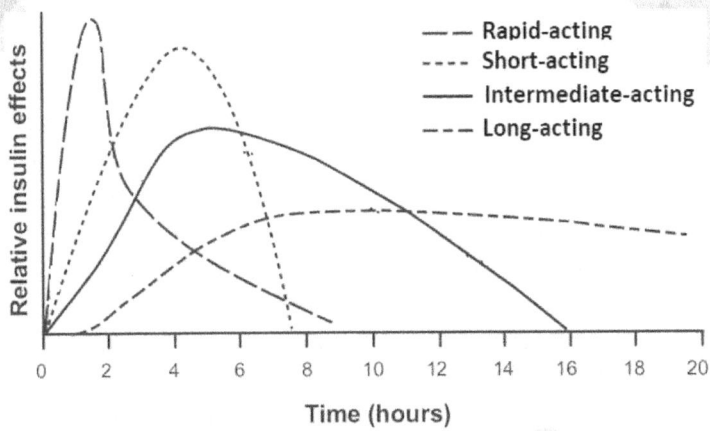

Time (hours)

Insulin types – duration of action

Type of insulin	Generic names	Onset | Peak | Duration [minutes]
• Rapid-acting	• Insulin aspart	15 | 30-90 | 180-300 min
	• Insulin glulisine	15 | 30-90 | 180-300 min
	• Insulin lispro	15 | 30-90 | 180-300 min
• Short-acting	• Regular insulin	30-60 | 120-240 | 300-480 min
• Intermediate-acting	• NPH	60-180 | 480 | 720-960 min
• Long-acting	• Insulin detemir	60 | no peak | 1200-1560 min
	• Insulin glargine	

At the initial stages when other glucose lowering agents are felt not to suffice in lowering glucose levels safely and effectively, addition of a basal insulin dose (NPH insulin or long-acting insulin analogue) to the patient's treatment regimen is a reasonable option. NPH insulin typically reaches peak activity 4-6 hours after injection, with its effects lasting 10-16 hours. Long-acting insulin analogues (insulin detemir, insulin glargine, insulin glargine U-300, insulin degludec) are peak less; their duration of action ranges from 12-16 hours for insulin detemir, 18-24 hours for insulin glargine, 24-28 hours for insulin glargine U-300 to 42 hours for insulin degludec). This approach is likely to suffice in patients with a shorter duration of diabetes, lower prevailing HbA1c and lower body mass index values.

At later stages of the disease, a twice- or four-times daily insulin regimen is required to achieve adequate glycaemic control. A typical twice daily insulin regimen would entail administration of premixed insulin before breakfast and dinner. A premixed insulin (e.g., Gensulin M30, Humulin M3, Mixtard) typically consists of a mixture of 70% isophane insulin and 30% soluble insulin. While having the advantage of fewer daily insulin doses, this insulin regimen is less flexible than that afforded by a basal insulin regimen but may be suitable for patients with a relatively fixed lifestyle. Premixed isophane/soluble insulin preparations are characterised by dual peaks at 2 and 6 hours, and a duration of action lasting 10-16 hours.

A basal bolus regimen requires the patient to receive a basal insulin and multiple short acting insulin preparations. Basal insulin (e.g., once/twice daily insulin glargine, twice daily insulin detemir, once daily insulin degludec, once daily insulin glargine U-300) aims to provide for basal insulin requirements, balancing glucose output by the liver. Basal insulin requirements are affected by body weight, stress, exercise, and alcohol. Three short acting insulin preparations (e.g., insulin aspart, insulin glulisine) typically administered shortly before /after breakfast, lunch and dinner are meant to cover for glucose excursions after meals. Insulin aspart and insulin glusiline typically reach peak activity 1-1.5 hours after injection, with clinical effect lasting 3.5 to 5 hours. Patients are trained to adjust their short acting insulin dose depending on the carbohydrate content of the meal and exercise, and to correct for prevailing pre-meal glucose levels (if elevated). The latter multi-dose insulin regimen is more physiologic and gives patients greater flexibility.

Psychological issues [1]

Introduction

A chronic illness or medical conditions are characterised by three main features: they are rarely cured, they do not resolve on their own, and they persist for a long time. This therefore necessitates that the individual resorts to frequent access to healthcare services. This continuing dependence on the healthcare services brings about psychological pressures, especially when the conditions appear in childhood and adolescence as often seen with Type 1 diabetes. When children are involved, psychological issues will also affect the parents and other family members. It is therefore essential for the affected individuals and their family members to be aware of the potential psychological issues which may arise so that they may be better geared to deal with them.

Reactive psychological stages

Chronic conditions can be characterised in two phases:

- phase one is the acute phase where the individual is diagnosed with the illness.
- phase two is characterised by a period of prolonged stress associated with long-term treatment, recovery, and survivorship.

Each phase will present the affected individual and their family with significant challenges and stressors that may have a major impact on the course of the illness. A diagnosis of a chronic condition brings with it the realisation that the illness is there for life, and while there are no prospects of a definite cure, the individual must undertake time-consuming, intensive, often tedious and inconvenient treatment tasks every day to manage the condition. Young people diagnosed with a chronic illness may have difficulty to accept their condition and providing treatment can be challenging for the healthcare professional. Moreover, every day, stress may be experienced on several levels: physically, emotionally, academically, or socially. This is because chronically ill children and adolescents are

---

[1] Prepared by Ms Stephanie Savona-Ventura.

confronted with uncomfortable symptoms, intrusive treatments, and further lifestyle restrictions such as physical limitations and diet. In addition, their chronic condition also may affect their school attendance and social activities. Furthermore, young patients suffering from a chronic condition may feel different from their healthy peers due to the significant lifestyle changes and stresses imposed on them by their medical condition. Depending on the condition involved, these lifestyle factors include issues such as increased healthcare attendances, the need to regularly use medications sometimes by injection, the need to constantly monitor diet and health sometimes using specific devices. All these factors may contribute to a poorer quality of life.

A diagnosis of any chronic condition elicits a psychological reactionary process emulating the Kubler Ross Stages of Grief. Grief occurs anytime an individual experience loss, in this case – loss of one's health. When diagnosed with diabetes, one often feels a loss of independence, or the loss of the opportunity to live life on one's own terms. Parents grief the loss of their "healthy" child and their child's healthy state of being. The grief process generally goes through five stages:

1. Denial: Living as if they are not affected with the condition, not caring what happens to them or how to move past the initial shock of the situation. While denial may be helpful in the short-term by postponing the fear and anxiety until the individual is in a better state of mind to cope with the psychological consequences of the illness, in the long-term denial may interfere drastically with adherence to treatment and self-management.
2. Anger: One may feel that their life quality potential has been tampered with and that additional restrictions have been imposed altering their lifestyle. Why me?
3. Bargaining: Bargaining with doctors, parents, family members, etc. trying to obtain agreement to their viewpoint of their condition.
4. Depression: Depressed sets in when the affected individual realises that all best laid plans to avoid accepting their affliction are not enough. The condition is there to stay.
5. Acceptance: The individual finally accepts the reality of the situation and the need to maintain regular glycaemic control. This level of acceptance fluctuates regularly.

The psychological reactions associated with the 'loss of health' grief process experienced by all patients after receiving news of the diagnosis is further compounded in adolescents. Adolescence development, even without the added pressures of a chronic illness, is itself characterised by stage-specific biological, psychological and social changes and adaptations.

A diagnosis of a chronic condition in childhood and adolescence can therefore potentially affect these developmental processes, while the physiological changes and psychosocial adjustments which form part of the adolescent developmental process can in turn affect the manifestations of the chronic condition. Adolescents of have adherence difficulties with diabetes management resulting in a deterioration in the overall metabolic control. The psychological factors that account for poor adherence are best understood within the context of normal adolescent development, i.e. experimentation, rebellion, risk taking, etc.

On a psychosocial level, adolescents initiate a process whereby they detach themselves from their parents, developing independence and becoming more involved with friends, i.e., emerge into adulthood. However, the emergence into the world of adulthood is not an easy process, and with this process comes a time of instability, anxiety, and insecurity as the individual finds his or her place in the community and the world. Adolescents diagnosed with a chronic illness will experience these normal developmental stressors, while simultaneously attempting to control and manage, as effectively as they can, their chronic illness. It is common for the individual, especially if in adolescence, to feel sad, lonely, anxious, and irritable. Outbursts of temper, pessimism about the future, and refusal to take insulin are less common responses and more cause for concern.

It is therefore clear that a chronic illness and the inconvenience of the management regimen can contribute to serve as a significant source of psychological stress for children, adolescents, and their families. This stress can contribute to emotional and behavioural problems that can consequently compromise adherence to treatment and medical advice. The family members, themselves undergoing the grieving process, out of fear and frustration, may feel compelled to motivate the adolescent with scare tactics. This may be counterproductive.

Psychological self-empowerment

It is essential that the individual suffering from any form of diabetes is helped to empower him/herself to deal not only with the long-term metabolic control, but also with the psychological facet of the disease process. The goal is successful diabetes management without letting diabetes interfere with the attainment of normal developmental tasks. This requires the individual to fully accept the condition and its life-changing consequences. Acceptance involves the balanced evaluation of the individual's illness and life, and the recognition for the need to adapt as is necessary. This is done by learning how to come to terms with the condition, to tolerate and handle the unpredictability of the disease

Once diagnosed with a chronic illness, the patient may react in a variety of ways.

1.   The individual may seek out support from others, exposing him/herself to positive interpersonal experiences that may strengthen the appreciation of relationships.
2.   By accepting their vulnerabilities and limitations, or by developing a heightened awareness of the fragility of life, the individual may develop a greater sense of personal resilience and strength, changing the way he/she views him/herself.
3.   The realisation that the illness may result in incapacity, or a shorter life can lead changes in priorities and values, and thus a change in the philosophy of life.
4.   The events of the chronic illness journey, whether positive or negative, will become part of a person's story about themselves.

The healthcare professional should take active steps to encourage this empowerment process by encouraging the patient and the family to label their respective concerns, to promote a collaborative relationship between the involved partners, and actively encourage shared decision-making in relation to designing management regimens. The patient and the family should feel encouraged to voice their concerns – there may be many misconceptions, fears and/or myths that need to be explored or acknowledged.

However, the strongest tool that helps to prepare the patients and family members to deal with the psychological issues is the provision of knowledge about the psychological processes in play. Being prepared for the normal reactions brought about by the grieving process will help the individual and his family to better adjust to living with the condition and this enable them to initiate an adjustment process and create a new normal by developing new priorities, reorganizing family responsibilities, renegotiating family relationships, and the integration of new routines.

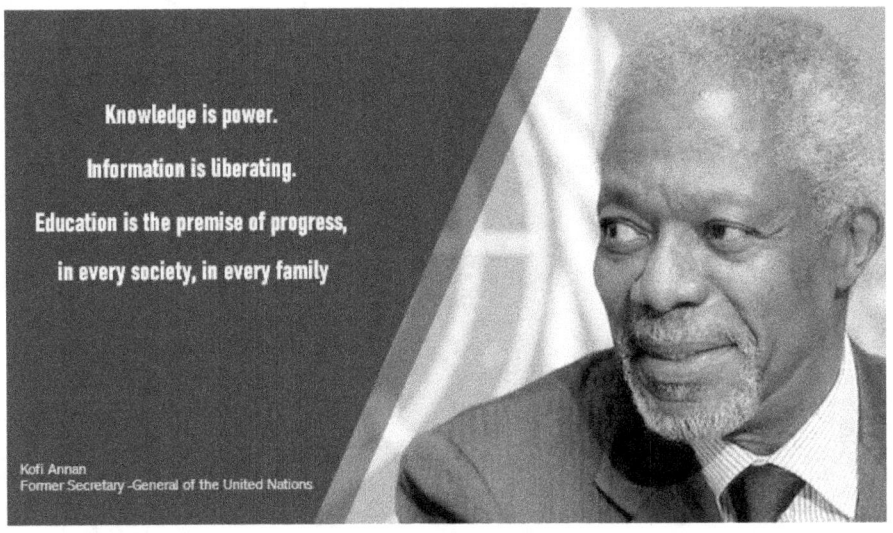

Knowledge is power.

Information is liberating.

Education is the premise of progress,

in every society, in every family

Kofi Annan
Former Secretary-General of the United Nations

Management in special circumstances [1]

Introduction

The diabetic person needs to be attentive in maintaining a close careful control of his/her metabolic state at all times and thus to adjust treatment regimens accordingly. The management may need day-to-day adjustments depending on the prevailing circumstances. There are particular situations where adjustments may become necessary since these circumstances may potentially significantly alter the metabolic state of the individual at that time.

Physical activity & Sports

Physical activity is an essential element in the management of diabetes. Moderate regular physical exertion during the course of the day or a planned daily episode of exercise should form part of the management of diabetes. If, however, one partakes in more vigorous competitive activity, then special precautions need to be taken to maintain a stable metabolic environment.

Diabetes should not be an impediment to competitive sports. Many individuals with diabetes take part in competitive sports and some have achieved international recognition. One of the best known ambassadors for diabetes in sports is the British athlete Sir Steve Redgrave (type I diabetes) who won a gold medal in rowing in five consecutive Olympic Games between 1984 and 2000. He was later knighted for his achievements. There have been many other athletes with both type I and type II diabetes who have been successful in their field both at national and international level.

---

[1] Prepared by Dr. Mario J. Cachia.

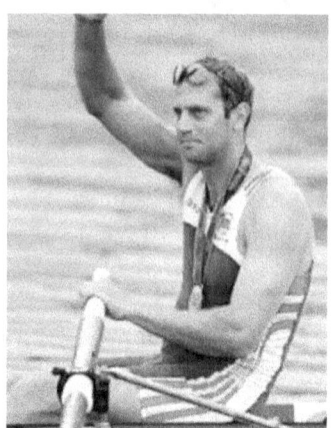

Sir Steve Redgrave wearing the Olympic Medal

Sporting activity places unusual demands on the body to produce energy at greater levels then is usual in the resting state. The production of glucose as an energy source for the body's needs is usually very dependent on the interaction of insulin and the liver, were most of the readily available carbohydrate is stored. This interaction results in a steady supply of glucose entering the blood stream to be transported to the various organs that require it for metabolism. In the resting state, most of this glucose is used up by the brain. When eating, the reverse tends to occur and the liver stores glucose as glycogen for later use.

Vigorous exercise, however, is an abnormal state for the body, mobilising a host of mechanisms which are aimed at increasing the efficiency of glucose utilisation and energy production. This leads to the body being able to use greater amounts of sugars and the use of other energy stores (such as fat) for metabolism. With exercise, the muscles are able to take up glucose more avidly and without a greater need of circulating insulin levels. This results from increased glucose flux to muscle cells due to an increased membrane levels of a transporter for glucose (GLUT4)[2] and the utilisation of any stored glycogen within the cells through the process of glycolysis. This mechanism may remain active for many hours after the

---

[2] GLUT4: glucose transporter which is able to take up glucose from the circulation, moves from the intracytoplasmic areas to the cell surface to transport glucose under the influence of insulin and exercise (mechanism unknown).

end of a vigorous bout of exercise. In persons who have diabetes, the period during and after exercise can be critical with a marked increase in the possibility of hypoglycaemic episodes for up to 48 hours.

Since the publication of the UKPDS and the DCCT trials[3], targets for control of blood glucose have become ever lower and the risk of hypoglycaemic episodes related to exercise is now greater then ever and can occur in both type 1 and type 2 subjects. It is therefore essential for persons with diabetes to be aware of their body's responses during various conditions and different types of exercise. In patients with type 2 diabetes not on insulin, it is often sufficient to take an extra small snack before exercise and perhaps another snack some time after the event. In type 1 diabetes or type 2 patients on insulin the situation becomes much more complex, partly because of the possibility of quicker onset of hypoglycaemia, but, also because of the use of longer acting basal insulin analogues which make dose alterations around exercise more difficult. The use of ultra-short acting insulin analogues, continuous glucose monitoring systems and pump therapy, has improved the outlook for people who undertake regular exercise.

Advice as to the dietary and therapy adjustments required during exercise have to be tailor-made both to the individual exercise and to the treatment regimen. Basic principles still apply as follows:

- Never exercise if unwell or significant urinary or blood ketones are present.
- Never exercise if hypoglycaemic. The optimal safe minimum glucose level at which to exercise will depend on a number of factors, but generally should not be below 8.0mMol/l. Some types of exertion which may cause severe hypoglycaemia or were hypoglycaemia can be dangerous (such as swimming), may require higher glucose levels pre-exercise.

---

[3] UKPDS: United Kingdom prospective diabetes study; a large UK based trial of optimum treatment in type 2 diabetes.
http://www.dtu.ox.ac.uk/index.php?maindoc=/riskengine/FAQ.php;
DCCT: diabetes control and complications trial, a large USA based trial in type 1 diabetes. http://diabetes.niddk.nih.gov/dm/pubs/control/.

- Some carbohydrate needs to be taken before exercise. A fruit or a cereal snack may be sufficient. Prolonged exertion may require carbohydrate intake at intervals during exercise. Suitable options would be small amounts of fruit juice or energy drinks.
- If multiple insulin injection regimens are used and exercise is planned, decrease the pre-exercise insulin.
- Significant increases in the daily amount of exercise, such as happens on a skiing holiday may require a decreased dose of basal long insulin. This is especially important for patients on the newer long acting analogue insulins which may require dose adjustments a couple of days before actually starting the holiday.

There is no doubt that exercise is an important aspect of the management of diabetes, and leads to improved glucose control and decreased cardiovascular risks. However there is surprisingly little scientific data as to the type, intensity and duration of exercise that is required to achieve a healthy lifestyle. What evidence there is points to the need for about half an hour of brisk exertion at least three times a week in adults. The definition of brisk exercise is also unclear, but perhaps an easy to follow rule is that with brisk exercise you get a sensation of mild shortness of breath. With this definition, a young person will need to work much harder then an older person. Also exercise intensity/duration will need to increase as one improves their fitness level.

Situations requiring significant dietary changes
1. Religious – Ramadan
During the Holy month of Ramadan, partaking of any food or drink during daylight hours for the whole lunar month is prohibited. Although those with health problems, including diabetes are exempt from fasting, many people with diabetes either do not regard their problem as an illness and hence do not expect to be exempt from fasting or are keen to fast as a sign of their faith. It is however prudent for people with diabetes to discuss the issue of the fast with a knowledgeable medical specialist who can guide them in advance so that any dietary and treatment modification can be planned. Patients who are on diet alone can usually adhere to the fast without any special precautions except to avoid overeating and eat a healthy diet. There is evidence that with sensible diet these patients can actually

lose weight and improve their glycaemic control. Patients who are on medications provide a more complex scenario. In the following table, various possibilities are briefly outlined, but each individual will need to be counselled for the particular medication.

• **Once daily oral sulphonylureas**
The morning tablet should be taken at dusk at the time of breaking the fast (Iftari).
• **Twice daily oral sulphonylureas**
Patients on twice daily oral agents should take the morning dose in the evening at the breaking of the fast (Iftari) and half the evening dose should be taken in the morning at the time of closing the fast (Sehri).
• **Three time daily oral sulphonylureas**
If patient is taking three times daily medication, then the midday dose should be omitted and the other medications adjusted as above. However, this may entail a change of medication, especially if patients are on long acting sulphonylureas.
• **Newer oral agents, metformin and injectable GLP-I analogues**
If patient is on the newer drugs and not on sulphonylureas, then minimal changes will be required.
• **Insulin**
As a rule, patients with type 2 diabetes who have been on long term insulin therapy or patients with type 1 diabetes should ideally not fast. However, if patients insist on fasting a long acting insulin analogue as a basal bolus to cover the daytime fast without actually causing hypoglycaemia should be used, supplemented either with plain insulin or better still with a short acting insulin analogue to cover the postprandial glucose peak and prevent hypoglycaemia a few hours after the meals. This regimen needs to be started in advance, so as to stabilise the patient prior to start Ramadan. The patients must always be advised that they need to monitor their blood glucose more frequently and that they should break the fast if hypoglycaemia occurs. For this purpose they should carry with them the usual emergency supply of sweets and carbohydrate.

It is also very important to recognise that each individual has different requirements and that changes to lifestyle and treatment have to be tailor-made to that particular individual's needs. Besides expertise in the management of diabetes, one needs to be able to discuss and plan with the patient well in advance so as to minimise the impact or if possible, benefit from this experience.

2. Other prolonged fasts and fasting for medical procedures.

a) *Prolonged fasting* for religious occasions other then Ramadan is now relatively rare, although some Christians still would like to fast on special days such as Good Friday. These fasts are different from that of Ramadan in that some persons fast for much longer periods, sometimes in excess of twenty-four hours. This makes it only practicable in persons who are well controlled on diet or on non-sulphonylurea oral hypoglycaemic agents. Blood glucose needs to be tested regularly during the period of fasting.

b) *Minor medical procedures and investigations:* Fasting for medical procedures is sometimes required. In the context of diabetes, fasting for blood letting is now hardly ever necessary and definitely not for cholesterol studies. When patients are required to fast, then the type of treatment, the duration of the fast and the procedure need to be taken into account. At most hospitals, guidelines are in place for most of these situations. Some general guidelines are discussed below.

- For patients on oral treatment, minor procedures such as gastroscopy, dilatation and curettage (D&C), minor foot surgery and others can usually be managed by omitting the morning medication and monitoring their diabetes on arrival at hospital. It is often possible to continue their medication for the rest of the day once the procedure is finished as there is only a short period afterwards were they are unable to eat or drink. As usual, blood glucose has to be closely monitored and if required an intravenous infusion can be set up to keep the glucose levels stable.

- Patients who are well controlled on conventional insulin should omit their treatment on the day of operation. They must be admitted early, started on an insulin, potassium and dextrose infusion and blood glucose monitored closely to enable adjustment of the insulin dose. Those on insulin analogues, should omit their morning short acting insulin and decrease (but not omit) the long-acting insulin.

- Patients whose diabetes is poorly controlled and are due for elective surgery, should have their diabetes reviewed and therapy adjusted as required. If the patient remains very poorly controlled then admission at least 24 hours prior to surgery is required.

c) *Major surgery:* Patients requiring elective major surgery should have their diabetes control optimised as much as possible prior to their operation. They should also be assessed for possible cardiovascular disease to avoid problems during surgery. Treatment should include continuous intravenous insulin. These patients usually require admission a day prior to surgery and if very poorly controlled, a discussion with a diabetologist is required. The infusion should be started late in the evening to allow a reasonable blood glucose by the morning. Patients should be continued on their pre-operative regimen until they are able to eat and drink, when they should be restarted on their previous treatment regimen. Regimens may need to be adapted to the specific circumstances of the patient and operation.

3. Dieting

Dieting for health or cosmetic reasons is now a common phenomenon. This is partly fuelled by the fashion industry, but also in part due to greater awareness that excessive body weight can cause health problems. Patients with diabetes should take weight reduction seriously as there is increased risk of cardiovascular disease. Patients must be aware that weight reduction necessitates calorie (and carbohydrate) restriction and therefore can lead to hypoglycaemia if improperly managed. Diets should be sensible. One should avoid quick diets; although these may work in the short term, the achieved weight loss is often regained rather quickly. Also extreme diets are much more likely to cause hypoglycaemia. Patients on metformin or the other non-sulphonylurea drugs usually require no change in medications. Patients on sulphonylurea agents will require a decrease in dosage. It is advisable that patients discuss major dietary changes with their diabetes specialist. It is important for patients to monitor their blood glucose levels regularly to avoid the risk of hypoglycaemia.

4. Parties and Festivities

Diabetes should not impede one from enjoying oneself. The patient with diabetes should try to live as much of a normal life as possible. Parties are unusual states of eating and drinking which often includes indulging in excess alcohol and occasionally also includes the intake of recreational drugs. In an ideal world one would eat and drink in moderation and perhaps increase ones medication slightly, especially if on insulin. However, since we live in the real world, situations of excess or abuse occur.

a) *Eating:* This discussion assumes that the parties occur late evening and the information also holds true to eating out in the evening. The intake of excessive amounts of calories especially in the form of carbohydrates should be avoided as should large amounts of fats. Since parties often last for several hours one should try to moderate food intake and spread this out over the whole time of the party. The food intake during the party should substitute the calorie intake of the closest meal. Treatment may need to be modified to prevent hypoglycaemia or severe hyperglycaemia. Subjects on oral hypoglycaemic agents should probably delay taking the tablets to just before the party. Patients on insulin therapy present a more complex situation. Patients on twice daily or multi-dose regimens should delay the evening dose of insulin to just before the party. Unfortunately, delaying the evening dose and the meal may result in either hypoglycaemia or hyperglycaemia depending on both the insulin regimen and the adequacy of glucose control. These situations can be avoided by knowing how your body would respond in these situations. If hyperglycaemia is the main problem, a small dose of a short or ultra-short acting insulin should be taken in the early afternoon together with a small snack. If on the other hand the problem is hypoglycaemia due to the effects of long acting insulins, then the solution is relatively straight forward as all that is required is a small snack in the early evening to avoid the hypoglycaemia. As usual all this advise needs to be tempered with regular and extra home monitoring.

b) *Alcohol:* In modern-day culture alcohol is synonymous with all sorts of celebrations and good food. Diabetes is not a barrier to alcohol consumption so long as moderation is adhered to. As a maximum, diabetics should not take more then 1-2 drinks per day.[4] Certain alcoholic beverages are better then others. The less alcohol and sugar a drink contains the more likely it is that blood glucose remains stable. Dry wines and light beers are good choices, as is diluting alcoholic drinks with sugar free mixers such as diet soft drinks. This has the added advantage of making the drink last longer, giving the liver more time to decontaminate the body and possibly also leading to decreased alcohol consumption.

Certain general guidelines also apply as listed below:
- regular meals should be taken and alcohol should not be consumed hours after any food intake[5]
- all diabetes medications should be taken
- always keep your blood glucose monitor with you and check frequently, especially if you are on insulin.
- always have treatment for low blood sugar with you. Remember that glucagon will not work if your hypoglycaemia is due to alcohol, as the liver will not be able to respond.
- Avoid exercise for a few hours before and after alcohol intake as this may further increase the risk of hypoglycaemia.

There are some situations were alcohol is best avoided altogether. These include:
- pregnancy and breast feeding
- driving and other activities were concentration or skill is essential
- certain medications, especially antibiotics such as metronidazole can cause reactions (flushing). There was also a diabetes medication (chlorpropamide) which can cause similar problems.
- if there are diabetes related complications such as neuropathy and retinopathy, as alcohol seems to accelerate deterioration of these problems.
- if there is hypertriglyceridaemia, as alcohol can further increase triglyceride levels.

---

[4] One drink means a tot of spirit, half pint beer or a glass of wine. Men should aim for less then 14 and women less then 9 drinks per week.
[5] Alcohol is metabolised in the liver in preference to glycolysis. As a consequence of this, 1 or 2 alcoholic drinks on an empty stomach can lead to very low blood glucose levels, especially in type 1 diabetes.

Alcohol excess can lead to serious complications. In addition to the problems with motor skill and judgement, alcohol excess can also lead to liver disease and deterioration in general health. This can eventually lead to serious liver disease with consequent ill health and early death.

Another problem with diabetes and inebriation is that the symptoms of hypoglycaemia can mimic or indeed coexist with the symptoms of drunkenness. This can lead to disorderly behaviour being attributed to alcohol causing delay in treatment of hypoglycaemia with potential for tragedy.

Chronic excessive alcohol intake especially in the context of malnutrition can also lead to problems in diagnosing acute diabetic ketoacidosis in type 1 diabetics. The usual scenario is of a patient looking very unwell, with dehydration, possibly altered mental state and abdominal pain. The blood glucose is tested and found to be less then 10 mmol/l leading to the erroneous assumption that diabetes is not the main problem. This scenario could easily be due to diabetic ketoacidosis, which is a medical emergency. This condition can be excluded by testing serum ketones .

5. Eating disorder

Patients with eating disorders are more vulnerable then most if they have diabetes, especially in type 1 diabetes. These are relatively rare conditions and only occasionally do we see such a case. Type 1 patients are the ones most likely to suffer as variations in foods intake will cause great shifts in glucose control and insulin requirement. There may be periods of hyperglycaemia, alternating with episodes of hypoglycaemia as the patients go from bulimia to anorexia. Some patients actually learn how to manipulate the dose of insulin, taking only enough to keep out of diabetic ketoacidosis but keeping themselves mildly ketotic at all times. This leads the body to use fat for energy and loose carbohydrate in their urine. These patients need intensive diabetes re-education in conjunction with psychological and psychiatric intervention.

6. Late nights

Everyone will on occasion require staying up late for an event. However, over recent years, the phenomenon of late weekends out, leaving home late in the evening and returning at around dawn has become a common phenomenon. These weekends are sometimes spent in entertainment establishments were diet drinks may be unavailable and water sold at a premium. During discussions with young adults, it seems that it is very difficult to go to any discothèque and eat or drink healthily. It is apparently the norm for these venues to offer alcohol and so-called energy drinks which are harmful to young people with diabetes. As one can surmise, the young adult with diabetes, who is almost certainly on insulin, has a number of obstacles to overcome in order to enjoy him/herself in such a fashion. Firstly there is the problem of changing the meal schedule and therefore the timing of the insulin doses, secondly there may be the problem of inappropriate meals and junk foods. Finally there is the problem of having the wrong type of drinks available. How one surmounts these obstacles will vary from person to person. It is probably best to discuss these problems with your specialists and try to work round them.

7. Recreational Drugs

Although 'recreational' drugs are generally considered illegal, their use is still a reality. Diabetic patients are no less subject to the use of these chemicals. There are very few statistics world wide on the use of these chemicals in diabetes. The use of some of these chemicals will pose potential serious effects on the person with diabetes.

a) Cannabis

Cannabis gives a feeling of light headedness, sickness, anxiety, depression and paranoid ideation. It can lead to psychological dependence, sensation of severe hunger which can cause problems with glucose control. It has effects on memory, leading to patients forgetting to take their insulin.

b) Cocaine

Cocaine is very addictive, leads to severe depression from dopamine effects on the brain. It is also a potent appetite suppressant. It has major cardiovascular effects with increased blood pressure and heart rate. It can lead to strokes, heart attacks and seizures. Due to neglect and lack of appetite, cocaine can be a cause for both hypoglycaemia and diabetic ketoacidosis.

c) Ecstasy (MDMA, 3,4-methylenedioxymethamphetamine)
Ecstasy effects the brain's serotonin system. It causes feelings of elation and happiness. However, its use has been shown to lead to long term brain damage in the neo-cortex and hippocampus. Its use has been associated with hyperthermia and dehydration leading to seizures and death. Diabetic subjects can seriously effect their health by using this drug.

d) Amphetamines
Amphetamines are mimickers of adrenaline, increasing short term drive and also increasing the metabolic rate. Amphetamines can lead to serious cardiac events if there is pre-existing heart disease which occurs at more frequently in diabetes. Patients with diabetes are at high risk of severe hypoglycaemia from increased metabolic rate and lack of appetite. After the effect of the drug wears of, patients may feel very hungry, resulting in hyperglycaemia.

If common sense and a sense of self preservation are completely lacking, then while reiterating the dangers prevalent in chemical abuse, a few precautionary issues should be highlighted. Eat plenty of carbohydrate in the form of pasta or potatoes and also bread to counter the effects of hypoglycaemia later. Take usual treatment. Drink plenty of non-alcohol fluids. Keep some form of identifying bracelet or keep some form of document to show you have diabetes. Take your meter with you and check your glucose levels often. Try to have a friend or partner who knows what to do in case of hypos (take sugar packets or fruit nectars).

Sexual Activity
The taboo and embarrassment surrounding sex can sometimes lead to problems for patients, partners and doctors. It is important to remember that a substantial portion of such problems are still related to anxiety and stress, even in the context of diabetes. Impotence is often the only sexual issue mentioned when one discusses the sexual complication of diabetes. This is perhaps due to its easy identification, however there are a number

of issues surrounding this topic which may be categorised in the following manner:

- Male sexual dysfunction
- Female sexual dysfunction
- Hypoglycaemia

1. Male Sexual dysfunction

Male sexual function can be effected by age, obesity, control of diabetes, duration of diabetes, medication and complications.

a) Erectile dysfunction

- Often when a man with diabetes complains of erectile dysfunction and impotence the blame is put squarely on diabetes. Diabetes is a common cause of impotence, however one must not forget that men with diabetes tend to have lower testosterone levels then normal and also they are not immune to other medical conditions causing impotence. Smoking and anxiety/stress are also common causes which may exacerbate mild organic erectile problems.
- The management of erectile dysfunction has been greatly simplified with the introduction of the phosphodiesterase type-5 inhibitors such as sildenafil, vardenafil and tadalafil. These drugs do have potential side-effects and drug interactions. Contraindications to taking these medications need to be carefully need to adhere to. These drugs are contra-indicated in patients on nitrate therapy and in patients were vasodilatation and sexual activity is inadvisable. They are also contra-indicated in patients with a history of ischaemic optic neuropathy. These drugs are also contraindicated in unstable angina, acute myocardial infarction, hypotension and recent stroke. These drugs are usually taken 30 to 60 minutes before sexual intercourse, although onset of effect may be delayed if taken with food, especially fatty meals. In diabetes, higher drug doses are often necessary.
- For those patients who do not respond to phosphodiesterase inhibition, few other options are available. Intracavernosal injection of prostaglandin E1 are reasonably effective but are only available with some difficulty on the local market. Recently, a new

system applying Prostaglandin E1 via the urethra has become available, but is not yet available locally.

- Another possible solution to impotence is the use of mechanical vacuum devices. These cause erection by creating a partial vacuum, which draws blood into the penis, engorging and expanding it. The devices have three components: a plastic cylinder, into which the penis is placed; a pump, which draws air out of the cylinder; and an elastic band, which is placed around the base of the penis to maintain the erection after the cylinder is removed and during intercourse by preventing blood from flowing back into the body. With the advent of orally effective medication, these devices are now much less popular as they are cumbersome to use and may cause pain.

- In refractory case, in young individuals, surgery may be considered as a final option. This necessitates the implantation of intracavernosal prosthesis of which there are two main types. The prosthesis is either a coil which is then inflated from a scrotal reservoir or the prosthesis is a flexible rod which the individual straightens to simulate an erection and achieve penetration. The main problem with these prosthesis is that they often cause ulceration and become exposed leading to a major surgical problem.

b) Retrograde ejaculation

- This occurs due to autonomic neuropathy[6] effecting the bladder and urethral sphincter. This results in the ejaculate being driven into the bladder rather then to the outside. In itself this does not cause medical problems, except if fertility is desired. Drug therapy (unlicensed indication) does not usually result in much improvement, imipramine or alpha-sympathomimetics (such as pseudo-ephedrine) may occasionally help.

---

[6] Autonomic neuropathy: damage of small nerve fibres which control such functions as bowel motion (nausea, vomiting, diarrhoea), bladder function (retention of urine), sweating, pupillary size.

c) Delayed ejaculation

- Delayed ejaculation in the context of diabetes is often related to delayed orgasm, at least in part due to decreased penile sensation. However, autonomic neuropathy also plays a role. Treatment is often unsatisfactory.

2. Female Sexual dysfunction

Up to fairly recently, the medical and diabetes textbooks had no mention of female sexual dysfunction induced by diabetes. Over the past decade or so this situation has become a much more prominent issue. It is still a difficult medical condition to diagnose and quantify, not least because patients do not often complain. It is known that women with diabetes have increased problems with achieving arousal and a decrease in sexual desire and increased difficulty in achieving orgasm. There seems to be no difference between diabetic and non-diabetic women having sexual dysfunction, until complications of diabetes start to develop.

Neuropathy is the organic cause for these problems in women. One issue is lack of vaginal lubrication and lack of increased blood flow to the genital areas on arousal due to autonomic neuropathy. Lubrication is relatively easily solved once recognised by use of lubricants, however blood flow cannot be restored with our present level of knowledge. The other problem is due to lack of sensation at the clitoris and vaginal wall. This will lead to problems in achieving orgasm. There is evidence that adequate control of blood glucose and blood pressure could lead to improved neurological function, so the possibility that sensation in this area returns is potentially available. There are of course other problems which can occur in women which are not due to diabetes itself, but in which diabetes plays at least a part. Problems with arousal can be due to problems with self esteem due to diabetes or due to other illness such as heart disease.

Drug therapy is unsatisfactory. Traditionally low dose androgens were used, but side-effects, especially hirsutism, makes them rather unpopular. Recently, some new drugs have been tested, showing some promise, but expense is a big limiting factor.

3. Hypoglycaemia and sexual activity

Sexual intercourse is a type of exercise and does lead to episodes of hypoglycaemia. It usually occurs in type 1 subjects and can effect both male and female patients. Patients are very distressed when this occurs since most would not have thought of this possibility and doctors and nurses tend not to mention sexual activity as a cause of hypoglycaemia. The management of this problem is the same as in any other cause of hypoglycaemia. It may be more problematic to prevent this as patients find it difficult to admit of the possibility of having to eat or drink prior or during a sexual encounter.

4. Contraception

All the various types of contraceptive methods that are in use by the general population can be used by the person with diabetes. The natural method, barrier methods, intra-uterine devices and male or female sterilisation pose no additional problems to the diabetic person. However, hormonal methods do raise concern in both patients and doctors. Most of these concerns arise from past experiences when high doses of hormones where used in the combined oral contraceptive pill (the pill). Modern dosage schedules have reduced the risks of major problems with this method. There is still a slight increased risk in the incidence of deep vein thrombosis and other blood vessel problems. In compensation, there is a decreased incidence of ovarian malignancy, decreased endometrial malignancy and a reduction of benign breast disease. Other hormonal methods include hormonal implants, which are becoming more popular. There is little if any evidence to suggest that diabetic women are more likely to suffer from the complications of these hormonal methods. However, it is prudent to keep one's blood sugar as normal as possible by self monitoring and HbA1c, avoid smoking and excessive alcohol intake and take regular exercise. It is also advisable to regularly check blood pressure as well as cholesterol and triglyceride levels.

Driving

Type 1 diabetes and type 2 patients on insulin are the ones who will mainly experience driving problems, although patients on tablets are not immune. This is due to hypoglycaemia. With tighter control targets for blood glucose, minor fluctuations can cause undetectable hypoglycaemia. Hypoglycaemia, even when mild and asymptomatic can cause cognitive impairment potentially leading to miscalculation and potential for accidents. EU regulations pose restrictions on the vehicles insulin treated subjects can drive. Maltese legislation does not appear to require the individual to inform the Police of any change in health status, except for severe hypoglycaemia – the law is reproduced below. A common sense approach would go a long way to prevent accidents while driving. You should not drive if you have recently been started in insulin, have eyesight problems, have neuropathy which interferes with the ability to hold the steering wheel and feel the pedals or you are unable to feel the early onset of hypoglycaemia. Many patients in Malta would not consider testing prior to driving, mainly due to a false sense of security due to short distances travelled. Many patients also find testing expensive and avoid testing. Recommendations for driving are listed below.

- Check your blood glucose before driving
- Do not drive if your blood sugar is below 3.8 mmol/l
- Make sure you have adequate supplies to correct hypoglycaemia. Ensure they are easily reachable.
- Never drink and drive, a cliché that holds more true for insulin treated as the risk of hypoglycaemia is increased.
- Recheck your blood glucose at regular intervals if driving for long periods (e.g. delivery drivers or driving holidays)
- If you do feel hypoglycaemic, stop the car at once and check.
- If hypoglycaemic, correct this and wait at least 30 minutes before driving again.
- Do not miss your appointed snacks because of driving.
- If you do get a hypoglycaemic episode, switch off the car and move off the drivers seat. In the U.K. patients having hypoglycaemic episodes have been charged with driving under the influence of a drug.

Diabetes Mellitus

6. In the following paragraphs, a severe hypoglycaemia means that the assistance of another person is needed and a recurrent hypoglycaemia is defined as a second severe hypoglycaemia during a period of 12 months.

Group 1:

(i) Driving licences may be issued to, or renewed for, applicants or drivers who have diabetes mellitus. When treated with medication, they shall be subject to authorised medical opinion and regular medical review, appropriate to each case, but the interval shall not exceed five years.

(ii) An applicant or driver with diabetes treated with medication which carries a risk of inducing hypoglycaemia shall demonstrate an understanding of the risk of hypoglycaemia and adequate control of the condition. Driving licences shall not be issued to, or renewed for, applicants or drivers who have inadequate awareness of hypoglycaemia. Driving licences shall not be issued to, or renewed for, applicants or drivers who have recurrent severe hypoglycaemia, unless supported by competent medical opinion and regular medical assessment. For recurrent severe hypoglycaemias during waking hours a licence shall not be issued or renewed until 3 months after the most recent episode. Driving licences may be issued or renewed in exceptional cases, provided that it is duly justified by competent medical opinion and subject to regular medical assessment, ensuring that the person is still capable of driving the vehicle safely taking into account the effects of the medical condition.

Group 2:

(iii) Consideration may be given to the issuing/renewal of Group 2 licences to drivers with diabetes mellitus. When treated with medication which carries a risk of inducing hypoglycaemia (that is, with insulin, and some tablets), the following criteria shall apply:

- *no severe hypoglycaemic events have occurred in the previous 12 months,*
- *the driver has full hypoglycaemic awareness,*
- *the driver must show adequate control of the condition by regular blood glucose monitoring, at least twice daily and at times relevant to driving,*
- *the driver must demonstrate an understanding of the risks of hypoglycaemia,*
- *there are no other debarring complications of diabetes.*
- *Moreover, in these cases, such licences shall be issued subject to the opinion of a competent medical authority and to regular medical review, undertaken at intervals of not more than three years.*

(iv) A severe hypoglycaemic event during waking hours, even unrelated to driving, shall be reported and shall give rise to a reassessment of the licensing status.

Maltese Legislation relating to driving licensing of diabetic individuals

Air travel

With the world becoming a smaller place and the recent introduction of no frills low cost long haul flights, air travel has become increasingly easy. Many patients with diabetes now undertake long flights, with problems of changes in length of day and delays potentially causing havoc with blood glucose control. Treatment adjustments are often only required for patients on insulin. The adage "westward=less insulin", "eastward=more insulin" often has to be tempered with a lot of common sense. There are some cardinal rules that must be observed when travelling:

- Visit your specialist or specialist nurse a good four to six weeks prior to departure to discuss any changes that may be required to your treatment regimen.
- Ensure you have adequate insurance cover. Make sure diabetes is covered.
- Ensure you take any required vaccinations and check if you need to take any insect repellents etc..
- Always take more medication then you require for your journey, especially insulin. Do not forget the delivery system (syringes, pens, needles etc.). Pack an insulin cool bag if travelling to a hot climate.
- With the heightened airport security, pack some form of identification to show you really have diabetes, especially if you have to carry insulin. Any insulin carried in the luggage (not ideal) should be packed in bubble wrap and then in thick clothes and packed in the middle of the suitcase. This is to prevent the insulin from freezing. On arrival the insulin needs to be checked for any crystal formation and if present discarded.
- Pack your glucose meter, lancets and strips, CGMS, pumps etc.
- Carry a note in the language of the country to say you have diabetes and which therapy you are having. Possibly also a note saying something like: I have diabetes, I am having a hypo, please give me some sugar.
- Keep all medical therapy in two separate bags, just in case one is lost or stolen.
- Check with the airline and also go on the website of the airports you are visiting to check for any changes in security.
- Always take plenty of extra carbohydrate, you may have to clear this with your airline well ahead of the flight.
- When travelling East:
  o Patients on conventional regimens (soluble insulin plus insulin isophane or insulin mixtures): it is probably easiest to take

73

conventional short acting insulin at regular intervals of about 5 to 6 hours and take a meal or a substantial snack at these times. This avoids problems with complex planning which can go wrong as soon as delays occur.

o   Patients on analogue insulins can continue their long acting insulin according to the interval they usually use and then take the short acting analogues with their meals and snacks.

o   Remember to test often, at least 4 hourly during your travelling

- Travelling West:

o   Patients on conventional insulins will need substantially less insulin for the perceived length of day. It is probably best to adopt a similar strategy to the one above, except that less frequent insulin will be required as the travelling day will be shorter. Avoiding the use of long acting insulin to prevent accumulation of insulin.

o   Analogue insulins are easier to manage. Work on keeping the long acting component at the required interval and take short acting analogues as required.

- Drink plenty of fluids on long haul flights and avoid alcohol.

- If you require insulin from the country of your holiday, be careful that the insulin is U100 (i.e. 100 units per ml). Some countries may still have availability of various other concentrations of insulin. This also holds true for delivery devices.

Scuba diving

Diabetes is usually considered a contra-indication for scuba diving. However, diet treated and type 2 patients not on sulphonylureas or insulin therapy should be able to dive safely as the risk of hypoglycaemia is minimal. Patients on sulphonylureas and those on insulin are usually considered not fit to dive although there tends to be more difficulty for patients on insulin. This is due to the perceived risk of hypoglycaemia and the difficulty in correcting hypoglycaemia under the sea. Recently some diving associations abroad have started to allow these people to dive if they meet strict criteria. These include the lack of any diabetes related complication, good control, lack of severe episodes of hypoglycaemia, no recent change in medication, no recent hospitalisation from diabetes related causes and a yearly medical check by a diabetologist [7].

---

[7] http://www.ukdiving.co.uk/information/medicine/diabetes.htm

Overall, it is recommended that until more information is available, it is safest for patients on insulin not to dive. However, since some patients would still opt to dive the following precautions should be taken (these precautions should also be taken by all who have diabetes):

- Try and keep your glucose control as stable as possible throughout the weeks and months around the time of diving.
- Do not even consider diving if you have had a recent unexplained hypoglycaemic episode.
- Check your blood glucose an hour before the dive then repeat half hour before and just before the dive. If there is a sudden drop do not dive. Do not dive unless blood glucose is stable and around 8 mmol/l. Try to change your insulin to the newer analogue insulin as these are less likely to cause unexpected hypoglycaemia.
- Carry some form of high calorie drink or paste which can be taken under water. Keep them in an easily accessible place.
- Make sure you never dive alone. Make sure that your diving companion knows how to deliver the drink or paste.
- Do not take extreme dives.
- Recheck your blood glucose as soon as you get out of the water.

Schooling

Children with diabetes should be able to enjoy the same schooling experience as any other children. Despite efforts to educate the educators, there is often resistance to treating these children as normal individuals. This unfortunately often leads to discrimination. There have been incidents were schools have asked for these children to be accompanied by a facilitator and frequent incidents were children were not allowed on school outings unless accompanied by their parents. What is worse, some of these children are expected to inject in the unhygienic environment of the rest rooms. Even in those schools were there is more understanding of the situation, these children are often not allowed to test their blood glucose or inject in class, even in an emergency. Occasionally we have also had cases were there children were not allowed to eat in class despite having hypoglycaemia.

When a child is diagnosed with diabetes, it is often the case that the parents believe this to be a major tragedy and tend to become over protective and in some cases try to hide the problems from everyone. Our first task as diabetes educators is often to allay this fear and help to develop a healthy relationship between the parents, the child and the environment including the school.

It is recommended that the parents visit the headmaster and explain the situation and if required we write letters or even have our specialist nurses visit the school. It is also suggested that close relatives and friends should be told about the diagnosis and some explanation about the condition given to them. Usually, those parents who encourage their children to hide their diabetes end up with children who are incapable of looking after themselves and may become rebellious teenagers. One often finds that close friends tend to be a stabilising influence rather then a disruptive one, reminding the child to watch his diet and drinks. This will also hold true for late teenage life were the children start going out and experimenting with alcohol etc.

Children should be taught how to manage their own diabetes as early as possible. Children as young as three years can start to inject and test their blood sugar, eventually taking control. The parents should try and play a supervisory role as early as possible so that the children become fully independent and so help to decrease the preoccupation of teachers and educators. A programmed injection schedule should be agreed with the specialist and the child encouraged to test at school, usually at midday break. Lunch breaks are important, and children should be encouraged to eat healthily. They should also be encouraged to participate in play during break times. It may be required to decrease the amount of insulin or increase the snacks on the day the children are going for their P.E. classes.

Employment
Patients without long term microvascular and macrovascular complications should be eligible for almost all jobs. There are a few jobs which the patient with diabetes is prohibited from undertaking. Most of these restrictions are related to insulin therapy, such as heavy vehicle driving and some jobs with the armed forces. However, most problems patients face, especially those treated with insulin, are related to ignorance and prejudice.

Again a sensible approach to choosing a job is called for. Jobs that are likely to be risky to life or limb should be avoided if the person is on insulin, especially if control is known to be erratic. Jobs that require climbing to heights (such as some crane drivers) or operate dangerous machinery (such as operating certain cutting tools) should be avoided by patients on insulin. If this is not possible then regular checking of one's blood glucose to avoid hypoglycaemia is required. Another consideration, again mainly effecting persons on insulin is working a shift system. Here the meal times and injection times as well as insulin doses may have to be adjusted on a daily or weekly basis depending on the type of shifts worked. As usual it is of utmost importance that these situations are discussed with your specialist and that blood glucose is monitored regularly. Here again, the use of the newer insulin analogues make control much easier as they allow a greater degree of flexibility.

The situation changes greatly once complications develop. The person with diabetes may have to give up his current employment and seek re-employment in a different category. For example, a stonemason would be unable to continue working if he suffers a heart attack. Complications may also lead to invalidity, for example a computer programmer who looses his eyesight or a taxi driver who suffers a stroke would obviously be eligible for invalidity pension.

Life Insurance
Insurance companies have over recent years become more restrictive in insuring patients suffering from diabetes. Patients are facing higher premiums on life insurance which young patients require to be able to take out a home or business loan. Some patients have had their premiums trebled and occasionally refused outright.

Diabetes and Adiposity in Pregnancy [1]

Introduction

Diabetes is a disorder in which the body does not produce enough insulin or does not utilise insulin properly. Insulin is a hormone that allows sugar to enter cells, where it can be turned into energy. In untreated diabetes, high levels of sugar can accumulate in the blood and damage organs, including blood vessels, eyes, and kidneys. Some individuals with diabetes need daily insulin injections to prevent these complications. The physiological changes that normally take place during pregnancy aiming to benefit the developing fetus will alter the way the pregnant women handle carbohydrate thus potentially altering significantly the metabolic control mechanisms of the diabetic mother.

Advances in the management of pregnancies complicated by diabetes and/or obesity have greatly reduced the risks involved and, today, most pregnant women with diabetes can look forward to having a healthy baby. However, it remains essential that the metabolic control in those with diabetes with or without accompanying obesity is closely maintained right through pregnancy to ensure the appropriate development and growth of the developing child and to reduce the medical risks from complications to the woman.

During pregnancy, two groups of diabetic conditions can be encountered:

- Pre-existing diabetes with/out obesity
- Gestational diabetes with/out obesity

Pre-existing diabetes

Women known to be affected by diabetes prior to their pregnancy can generally be grouped into those women who have Type 1 diabetes and those who have Type 2 diabetes. There are further patients who are

---

[1] Prepared by Dr. Johann Craus & Prof. Charles Savona-Ventura.

diagnosed to have monogenic forms of diabetes giving rise to Maturity-Onset Diabetes of the Young (MODY) and other specific types of diabetes. Since Type 2 diabetes is usually seen in relatively elderly individuals, the commoner form of diabetes seen during pregnancy is generally Type 1 diabetes, though the increasing predisposition to delaying one's reproduction and increasing predisposition to obesity in the developed world has resulted in an increase in the prevalence of Type 2 diabetes seen during pregnancy. These individuals are usually diagnosed and being managed prior to them embarking on a pregnancy experience. Because of the potential risks of complications to the developing child and the woman, it is particularly essential that very close metabolic management is achieved throughout the pregnancy starting even before embarking on the pregnancy journey.

Women with poorly controlled pre-existing diabetes in the early weeks of pregnancy are several more times likely than the non-diabetic women to have an infant with serious birth defects, such as a heart defect or a neural tube defect affecting the spinal cord or brain. They also are at increased risk of miscarriage and stillbirth. Women with poorly controlled diabetes are also at an increased risk of having a very large macrosomic baby. The babies of poorly controlled diabetic mothers grow excessively because the extra maternal sugar in the mother's blood crosses the placenta and goes to the fetus. The fetus then produces extra insulin to help process the sugar converting this into fat. The fat thus produced tends to accumulate around the shoulders and trunk, sometimes making these babies difficult to deliver vaginally and putting them at risk of injuries during delivery. During the new-born period, babies of all women with poorly controlled diabetes are at an increased risk of breathing difficulties, low blood sugar levels and jaundice. While these problems can be treated and managed when identified, it is better to prevent their occurrence by keeping a very good control of blood sugar levels during pregnancy.

The main maternal complications of pre-existing diabetes are generally related to the two extremes of poor control, namely a hyperglycaemic crisis [high blood sugar] and hypoglycaemic episodes [exceedingly low blood sugar]. Both situations can be detrimental to the health of the mother, though hypoglycaemia is generally considered the more dangerous situation since this can result in a sudden maternal death. Both situations

80

have consequences on the developing child, consequences that can lead to its death in utero. The women with a hyperglycaemic crisis will become acidotic resulting in a significant alteration in the overall metabolic environment. These changes are transmitted to the fetus-in-utero leading potentially in its sudden death. During a hypoglycaemic episode, the low blood sugar in the mother is closely reflected in the blood sugar levels of the fetus-in-utero potentially also leading to its sudden death or stillbirth. The diabetic mother is also at risk of other pregnancy complications including a higher rate of spontaneous miscarriages, pregnancy-related hypertension, and polyhydramnios [an excess of amniotic fluid] which can contribute to premature labour and problems with fetal presentation during labour. The pregnancy can also augment the general effects caused by the diabetic state which can damage organs such as the eyes, kidneys, and blood vessels.

In the light of these potential serious complications, it is crucial that known diabetic women embarking on a pregnancy are very closely monitored and controlled to reduce the risks to the woman and the developing child. With appropriate medical care and obstetric management, the outcome should be very favourable so that the obstetric outcomes of the diabetic mother are equivalent to those of the non-diabetic one. In the year 1989, the St. Vincent Declaration included, among its aims, a target for the pregnant diabetic individual whereby the aim was set "To achieve pregnancy outcome in the diabetic woman that approximates that of the non-diabetic woman". However, for a woman with diabetes who is pregnant, or who plans to become pregnant, intensive management of diabetes is critical. Diabetes control is important both before and after conception to ensure the health of the mother and the unborn child.

Preconception Care: Women with pre-existing diabetes, whether Type 1 or Type 2 DM, planning to embark on a pregnancy should consult their doctors before the pregnancy to ensure that their blood sugar levels are well controlled. This is important because the most serious birth defects associated with diabetes originate in the early weeks of pregnancy, before a woman may realise, she is pregnant. It has been repeatedly shown that blood sugar control begun prior to pregnancy largely eliminates the extra risk of birth defects for women with pre-existing diabetes requiring insulin. Other studies show that blood sugar control before and during pregnancy reduces the risk of miscarriage, stillbirth, macrosomia, and complications in the new-born period.

Before embarking on a pregnancy, the woman with diabetes should ensure that her health is as optimal as is possible and embark on a series of interventions to reduce the risks to her planned pregnancy. In the meantime, it remains essential to continue using a contraceptive method until the clinical condition is deemed sufficiently controlled to be considered optimal for pregnancy initiation. In conformity to all women embarking on a pregnancy, the diabetic individual should ensure that they have been immunized against Rubella (German Measles). The status of immunization can be checked by a simple blood test; and if immunity has not been previously achieved, then vaccination should be requested.

Some medications, including tablets taken to manage a high blood pressure or to lower cholesterol, may have a deleterious effect on the developing embryo. The opportunity should also be taken at this stage to review the general health of the diabetic woman, including an assessment of renal function and an ophthalmologic examination. Any abnormalities noted should be addressed prior to embarking on a pregnancy since the pregnant state can predispose to a deterioration of these conditions. Smoking is generally harmful to health and has specific effects on the developing foetus. It should therefore be stopped completely during this period.

The pregnant woman should also ensure that her dietary intake includes a high proportion of fruit and vegetables to increase the intake of antioxidants. Antioxidants are vital for cells to survive and combat the harmful effects of "free-radicals". These "free radicals" are produced at increased rates in the presence of hyperglycaemia and adversely affect embryonic development causing the early miscarriages and malformations. In addition, it is important to take regular Folic Acid supplements for at least 3 months before and for the first 3 months of any pregnancy. Women with pre-existing diabetes are at increased risk of having a baby with a Neural Tube Defect, so taking folic acid is especially crucial for them since this has been shown to reduce the chances of having a child with these defects. For a mother with diabetes, 5mg tablets are usually prescribed rather than the 0.4 mg tablets advised for women without diabetes.

The most essential aspect of preconception care of the diabetic woman is to ensure a rigid blood glucose control. The diabetic woman wishing to embark on a pregnancy should ensure that her blood glucose is as near to normal as possible for at least 3 months before becoming pregnant. This means that the blood glucose targets should aim at a level of 4-6 mmol/l before meals and no higher than 8 mmol/l when tested two hours after a meal. Long-term control of the diabetic state is usually assessed by the glycosylated haemoglobin test (HbA1c). The target should aim at an HbA1c level of less than 7 percent before becoming pregnant.

The attending physician may also need to review the diabetic treatment being used.
- If the diabetes is treated with insulin, then there may be the need to change the insulin doses or even change the number of injections taken during the day.
- If the diabetes is treated with oral hypoglycaemic tablets, then the physician may prefer to replace these with insulin injections and obtain good control before the pregnancy. While some oral hypoglycaemic have been shown to be safe during pregnancy, not all forms have been fully evaluated and confirmed as being safe to use.
- If the diabetes is managed by diet alone or in obese women, then it may be prudent to review the actual current metabolic situation before pregnancy with appropriate investigations [e.g., an oral glucose tolerance test] to ensure that appropriate management is being given.

Any changes in medication may cause a transient loss of control in the medical condition being treated, and it thus is essential that this control is regained prior to embarking on the desired pregnancy.

Antenatal management: Once a pregnancy is diagnosed, usually at around five weeks after the last menstrual period, it is important to arrange an early visit to the obstetric and diabetic team. Now, it is imperative that

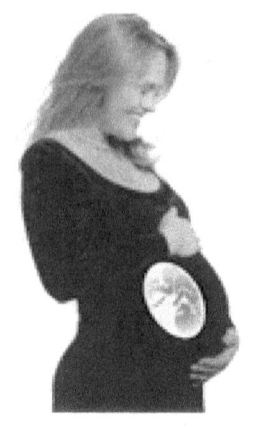

the blood glucose is maintained as near to normal as possible throughout the whole of the pregnancy. This may not always be easy and needs regular modifications to the metabolic regimen since the physiological changes of pregnancy result in alterations in the body's response to and needs for insulin. Metabolic control is primarily based on dietary modifications, and alterations in hypoglycaemic agents' dosage, particularly in those women on insulin. Towards this aim, the attending physician may require the woman to test her blood glucose more frequently ideally before and after each meal and before bedtime, but extra tests may also be necessary. Self-monitoring of blood glucose with a reliable system is the optimum. For good control, the blood glucose should be kept as close to normal as possible, while avoiding hypoglycaemia. The scope of therapy [diet +/- insulin] is to maintain a fasting and after meal glucose levels of <5.5 mmol/l and <8.0 mmol/l respectively. Long-term control can also be assessed regularly during pregnancy by measuring glycated haemoglobin [<8.0%] or fructosamine, aiming to achieve levels within the normal non-diabetic range.

Dietary advice is essential for optimal diabetic control during pregnancy. All women who have diabetes should have regular access to a dietitian. Dietary advice should be individualized on the basis of the woman's weight, home blood glucose monitoring, lifestyle and personal circumstances. Food intake should be adequate to maintain maternal and fetal nutrition. An energy prescription of 30-35 kcal/kg pre-pregnant ideal body weight is recommended, though this should be flexible to correct for any alteration in activity levels. Those women whose body weight exceeds 120% of their ideal body weight may require a lower energy intake per kg in order to limit their weight gain during pregnancy. Frequent small meals may facilitate improved blood glucose control. Exercise remains an essential feature of maintaining the woman's

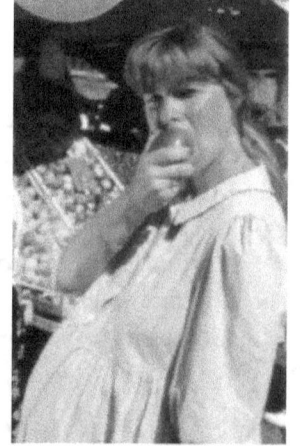

wellbeing. Complex carbohydrates should provide about 50% of the total calories. This should be distributed in the form of 10-gram exchanges as regular main meals and snacks throughout the day. Levels of dietary fibre of 30-50g per day should be advised. Foods rich in antioxidants - fresh fruits and vegetables - may have a role in reducing malformations. All foods containing refined sugars, e.g., cakes, ice-cream, sweets, soft drinks, should be strictly avoided preferably by all pregnant women irrespective of their carbohydrate metabolism status. Folate supplements (5 mg/day) should be routinely prescribed in the first trimester to reduce the risk of neural tube defects.

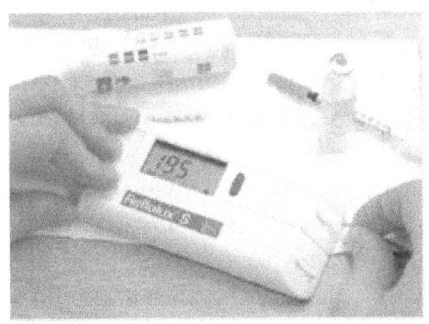

To achieve this good control, alterations in the medical management including extra insulin injections for those women on insulin or the introduction of insulin treatment for those on oral hypoglycaemic tablets are generally required. The overall insulin requirements will increase after 20 to 24 weeks and stabilise by about 36 weeks. It is not uncommon for a woman on insulin to require her to take around 3-5 times her usual daily non-pregnant dose - this is normal. Once the baby is born, the dose will return to the pre-pregnancy levels. Insulin regimens should be individualized. It is usually preferable to use human insulin in the form of multiple injections of short-acting insulin with long or intermediate-acting insulin at night. Alternately, twice daily, short and intermediate-acting insulin may be appropriate. Estimation of insulin requirements can only be gauged after metabolic daily blood glucose profiles have been obtained. The initial requirements can follow the administration of short-acting insulin according to a sliding scale, the dose depending on the blood glucose level [see table below]. The daily requirements can then be assessed and managed by the introduction of intermediate acting insulin.

	BLOOD GLUCOSE LEVELS	MANAGEMENT
INSULIN SLIDING DOSE	➤ 10.0-12.2 MMOL/L	➤ 4 UNITS
	➤ 12.2-13.3 MMOL/L	➤ 6 UNITS
	➤ 13.3-15.6 MMOL/L	➤ 8 UNITS
	➤ 15.6-16.7 MMOL/L	➤ 10 UNITS
	➤ 16.7-18.9 MMOL/L	➤ 12 UNITS
	➤ >18.9 MMOL/L	➤ 14 UNITS

Insulin sliding dose scheme

During pregnancy, it is not uncommon to experience hypoglycaemic events more frequently. Pregnancy unfortunately will also alter the normal warning symptoms of hypoglycaemia thus potentially reducing the woman's perception of an oncoming episode. It is important for the diabetic woman on insulin to be careful about driving, sleeping through snacks or spending long periods of time alone. If the woman is experiencing frequent hypos, then it may be wise to stop driving altogether until the metabolic control is readjusted and stabilized. Standard tests to check the status of the eyes and kidneys should be performed at least three times during the pregnancy – once every trimester. Further attention is given to diabetic women to assess maternal and foetal well-being throughout their pregnancy to identify signs of foetal compromise early and institute timely intervention.

Long-term diabetes mellitus with its attendant hyperglycaemia and hyperinsulinaemia causes significant damage to the various body organs, particularly the eye retina and kidneys. The metabolic imbalances promote the proliferation of poorly structured blood microvessels which are evident in the retina in the form of retinopathy. These changes will in the long-term result in blindness. The kidney microstructure is also affected by long-term diabetes mellitus resulting in chronic renal failure. Pregnancy causes profound changes in the various organs of the body; primarily aimed at promoting foetal growth and well-being. However, these changes may accelerate the complications generally associated with diabetes mellitus with the development of proliferative retinopathy and nephropathy. Diabetic women embarking on a planned pregnancy should ideally have a pre-conception check of the eyes and kidneys to ensure that these organs are in optimal health. During the pregnancy, these organs should be rechecked clinically and biochemically at three monthly intervals to identify early the development of complications and institute timely treatment.

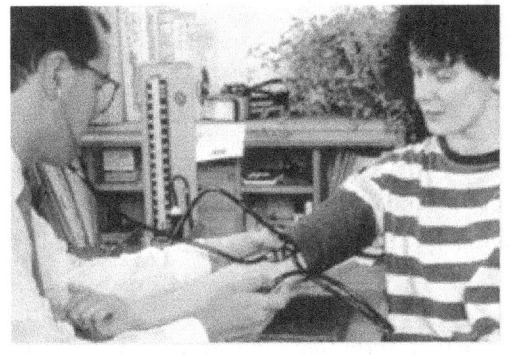 A major complication of pregnancy that has a significant maternal and foetal morbidity and mortality rate is that of pregnancy-induced hypertension and pre-eclampsia. This condition, typified by multiorgan disease damage, is more likely to occur in women suffering from diabetes. The possible development of this initially insidious disorder or pregnancy, identifiable by a rise in blood pressure and the development of albuminuria, requires the close monitoring of pregnant diabetics with more regular antenatal visits.

The Obstetric team would also assess and review the pregnancy more intensely to assess the well-being of the developing child. Clinical assessment at every antenatal visit remains critically important. This requires regular assessment of uterine size correlated to gestational age, foetal wellbeing through foetal heart auscultation, blood pressure measurement, body weight, urine analysis for glucose and protein, and assessment of foetal presentation and engagement in the last trimester. The assessment of foetal movements by the mother herself during the third trimester may have a role in the management of diabetic pregnancies identified as high risk.

However, ultrasound scanning forms the basis of surveillance of the foetus of the diabetic woman to confirm gestational age, exclude congenital malformations, assess foetal growth, and foetal wellbeing. An early scan in the first trimester helps confirm the gestational age through the measurement of crown-rump length. A repeat scan at 18-22 weeks gestation further confirms the gestational age through the measurement of biparietal diameter and other criteria. This latter scan also examines for the presence of congenital anomalies. Serial ultrasound measurements from the late second trimester onwards, using foetal growth parameters including circumference measurements of the abdomen and head are essential to determine normal foetal growth and identify early asymmetric growth acceleration or deceleration. Foetal weight estimates in cases of suspected excessive growth may help in decision-making about mode of delivery. These third trimester growth assessment scans are coupled with assessments of foetal wellbeing.

There is no single reliable test for the assessment of foetal well-being and attention should be targeted at the particular pathology which is suspected. Women with vascular disease and hypertension may have relatively early onset intrauterine growth retardation. Babies of such mother are at very high risk but standard testing with Doppler and biophysical monitoring is likely to be predictive of intrauterine growth retardation and foetal compromise. Serial foetal biophysical profiles based on a modified Manning Score using ultrasonography and cardiotocography are advised. The modified Manning Score below takes into account the presence of increased liquor volume since this may be a sign of inadequately controlled carbohydrate metabolism. Foetal compromise may result from an imbalance between placental function and foetal metabolic demands, such as occurs in macrosomic babies with polyhydramnios. The predictive power of biophysical monitoring for this type of metabolic-based compromise is of short duration. The timing of starting and the frequency of testing must depend on the risk assessment. However, once to twice weekly monitoring starting at 36 weeks gestation may be considered a reasonable practice, with an earlier onset in the presence of poor diabetic control, vascular disease, or abnormal foetal growth.

Management during delivery: During the last month of pregnancy a decision about the eventual mode of delivery is made. Though women with diabetes are at increased risk of caesarean delivery because of the association with large babies, most can have a normal labour and vaginal delivery. The aim is generally to try to achieve a normal labour and delivery whenever possible and whenever this is considered a safe option for the infant. The timing of delivery should therefore be individualized depending on whether the pregnancy is associated with any significant complications of the diabetes such as very poor metabolic control, any complications of pregnancy such as hypertensive or renal disease, and on the size and well-being of the foetus. It should theoretically be possible in a woman with good diabetic control and no obstetric or diabetic complications to continue the pregnancy to term [39-40 weeks], but definitely not further than the calculated expected date of delivery. There is no evidence that prolonging pregnancy beyond this date is beneficial, while there is some evidence that delay may be detrimental by increasing the risks to the infant.

Sometimes, if the infant is assessed to be macrosomic [overweight], or if there is poor diabetic control, or if the blood pressure goes up, or if there is evidence of insufficiency of the placenta; the obstetrician may wish to deliver the child earlier. This early intervention may bring about possible infant complications related to prematurity, particularly of problems with respiration. In the past, foetal lung maturity was assessed in these situations by means of amniocentesis and the measurement of amniotic fluid surfactant levels prior to delivery of a diabetic pregnancy. This is today no longer required with a delivery after 38 weeks, and it should rarely be needed even at an earlier gestation. The administration of prenatal steroids for twenty-four hours prior to the elective preterm delivery can be considered since this may help optimise foetal lung maturation. However, steroids increase insulin requirements and judicious use is essential since the administration of this medication may further tip the balance in respect to metabolic control and bring about ketoacidosis to the detriment to the mother and child.

Preterm labour may also occur spontaneously. The management of preterm labour includes the option of using medications which reduce uterine activity, generally with the aim of gaining at least twenty-four hours to enable the administration of steroids to accelerate lung maturity and decrease the foetal risk of respiratory distress. These uterine depressant medications however may have pronounced hyperglycaemic effects and are best avoided in the diabetic woman. If deemed necessary, then very judicious use can be made of this medication, usually combined with steroid administration for twenty-four hours, and very careful monitoring of blood glucose levels and the administration of insulin according to requirements.

Early timed delivery can be achieved either by performing an elective Caesarean section; or by inducing labour medically using prostaglandin [a medication that helps soften the uterine cervix in preparation for labour], followed by an oxytocin intravenous infusion [a medication that brings on contractions] with artificial rupture of membranes [a procedure that also stimulates the onset of labour]. The procedure of induction of labour may be undertaken according to the normal regimen used for non-diabetic women, except that the oxytocin infusion must be diluted in a saline solution rather than the usual dextrose [a type of sugar] solution. During the preparation of the cervix with prostaglandins, the diabetic woman can maintain her normal diet and dose of insulin. However, with rupture of the membranes and/or the initiation of an oxytocin infusion, the diabetic woman must be managed with a strict regimen to maintain metabolic control.

The intrapartum management requires very careful attention to prevent either hypoglycaemia or ketoacidosis, and thus necessitates the maintenance of the blood glucose levels to as near normal as possible. Unless the diabetic insulin-dependent woman has a very rapid spontaneous labour, it will be necessary to administer intravenous insulin and dextrose to prevent ketoacidosis or hypoglycaemia. An intravenous infusion of dextrose containing potassium salt is generally set up to run at a rate of 500 millilitres every four hours. Into this drip, a motorized syringe is set up to inject a continuous dose of insulin. The insulin dosage is adjusted according to the hourly blood glucose values. Potassium levels should be checked at admission and every six hours aiming to maintain levels of 3.4-4.8 mmol/l. Any oxytocin administered to augment the progress of labour should be given in an infusion of saline solution via a separate infusion pump.

Effective pain relief is important, and all forms of pain relief used in labour can be used. Pre-loading saline infusions necessary when setting up an epidural should be administered via a separate intravenous access than the glucose-insulin infusion. The foetal heart rate should be continuously monitored throughout labour and delivery. The possibility of the baby being very large and causing mechanical problems should always be considered. Size may be underestimated both clinically and by ultrasound, and problems with the delivery of the shoulder [dystocia] in diabetic pregnancies occurs at lower birth weight than in non-diabetic pregnancies. Where the baby is thought to be large but vaginal delivery is planned, slow progress should always prompt consideration for Caesarean section. Experienced obstetric staff should be present for vaginal delivery and must be prepared to deal with shoulder dystocia. In all cases the paediatrician must be alerted to be present at the time of birth.

Insulin-dependent women undergoing elective Caesarean section should be managed with an intravenous dextrose drip and insulin pump started on the morning of the operation and continued postoperatively until the woman is able to take fluids by mouth and is able to eat without vomiting. The Caesarean section should ideally be performed the first thing in the morning. Breakfast and the morning insulin dose is omitted and the dextrose/insulin regime started about one hour before the surgery. If the operation is scheduled for the afternoon, then a light breakfast and quick-acting insulin [e.g., Actrapid or Humulin R] is given in the morning. The dextrose/insulin regimen is started about one hour before the surgery or around noon. Blood glucose is monitored every hour in the post-operative period and the insulin dose adjusted accordingly.

Management after delivery: The metabolic requirements change drastically after delivery, and insulin requirements fall dramatically. Occasionally no insulin may be required for a few hours. The insulin dose in insulin-dependent diabetic women should be reduced to about the pre-pregnancy level - however these women should be encouraged to run their blood glucose levels slightly higher than they did during pregnancy because of the danger of becoming hypoglycaemic while handling the baby; but also, they must be encouraged not to neglect their diabetic care because of the increasing demands of their new family. Women who require intravenous feeding postpartum, e.g., after a Caesarean section, should have their insulin infusion rate decreased to half their intrapartum requirements.

If the infant had been very large [macrosomic] or there had been evidence of excessive amniotic fluid [polyhydramnios], the mother particularly if multiparous is at greater risk of postpartum haemorrhage. Prophylactic measures are generally taken to prevent postpartum haemorrhage, including the routine administration of intramuscular syntometrin® and followed by a continuous infusion of the uterine stimulant oxytocin in a saline infusion for the first 12 hours postpartum. Prophylactic antibiotics should be given if the delivery was by Caesarean section.

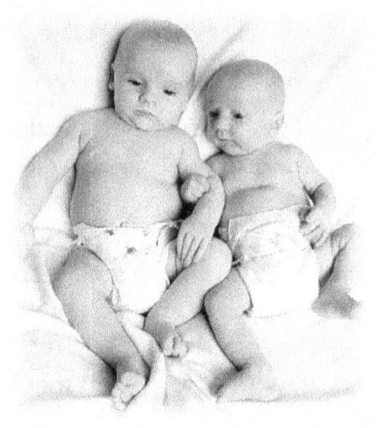 A paediatrician skilled in resuscitation of the new-born infant should always be present during the delivery of women with diabetes. Babies born to insulin-dependent diabetic mothers nearly always go to the Neonatal Intensive Care Unit for a short period of observation because of the higher risks of neonatal complications arising from hypoglycaemia. Hypoglycaemia or very low blood glucose levels is a frequent problem in infants of diabetic mothers resulting from the fact that the foetal pancreas was accustomed to an increased rate of insulin secretion during intrauterine life. Hypoglycaemia can have devastating effects of the infant if unrecognised and untreated. The blood glucose of the new-born infant should be measured frequently during the first 24-48 hours, though the exact timing of the sampling is controversial. An early glucose feed in these infants is generally indicated to prevent the complication. The problem of hypoglycaemia is more likely to occur in the premature infant, since the nutritional stores of the child are not necessarily well developed. The premature infant of the diabetic mother is also more susceptible to complications generally associated with prematurity, such as respiratory distress, low calcium blood levels, poor liver function causing hyperbilirubinemia, and convulsions. All these problems would require specialized neonatal care hence the need for a period of observation in the Neonatal Intensive Care Unit for those infants considered at increased risk.

Breast Feeding is encouraged; but until lactation is well established, formula or glucose feeds will be necessary to prevent hypoglycaemia in the infant. Breast milk is very rich in carbohydrates, and thus the nutritional demands require an increased intake of starchy foods to make up for this increased loss. In addition, the dose of insulin required may be reduced while breastfeeding since the baby is taking significant amounts of carbohydrate from the mother. The insulin-dependent diabetic mother should test her blood glucose before and after breastfeeding to enable her to correctly adjust the insulin and food intake.

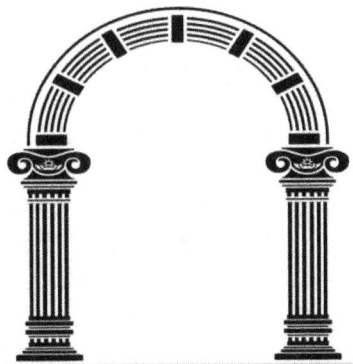

Diet & lifestyle	Metabolic control
• Encourage diets with high levels of complex but not refined carbohydrates and soluble fibre and reduced saturated fats. • Promote fresh fruits and vegetables. • Folic acid supplements should be offered. • Promote exercise, at least 30 minutes' walk each day.	• Use of multi-dose insulin injections and intensified self-monitoring of blood glucose. • Maintain blood glucose levels of 4-6 mmol/l before meals and under 8 mmol/l two 2 hours after meals. Ensure an HbA1c level of under 7%. • Checks for ketonuria should be made if blood glucose is high or in the presence of intercurrent illness.

- The eye retina, blood pressure and renal function should be assessed regularly.
- Ultrasound scanning must be made available for assessing gestational age, examining for congenital anomalies and for assessing fetal growth.
- Maternal monitoring of fetal movements should be encouraged. Fetal monitoring with cardiotocography and biophysical profiles is controversial, but it should definitely be used for high-risk pregnancies.

Principles for managing the pre-existing insulin-dependent diabetic mother during pregnancy

Gestational diabetes

Gestational diabetes [GDM] usually presents as a transient disorder identified during pregnancy but the condition resolves once the pregnancy ends. It is brought about by the physiological changes engendered by the pregnancy. It usually presents and is diagnosed in the third trimester of pregnancy. However, there are individuals who may have been undiagnosed diabetics or have sub-clinical pre-diabetes [impaired glucose tolerance - IGT] prior to the pregnancy and are only diagnosed as a result of the screening that occurs during the pregnancy – Diabetes in Pregnancy [DIP]. It is therefore essential that women at risk of developing diabetes are encouraged to seek pre-conceptional care so that they can be assessed as to their metabolic state and to ensure that they are not already suffering from a latent form of the disorder. Before pregnancy, weight loss is advised to those with excess body weight from their correct weight range and height. However, weight loss is unadvisable once pregnancy is started.

- Women aged more than 35 years.
- Obese individuals with a Body Mass Index ['BMI] >30 km/m².
- Women who have features of polycystic ovarian disease syndrome including irregular, delayed and anovulatory menstrual cycles.
- Women with a family history of diabetes especially maternal and siblings.
- Women with a past history of gestational diabetes in a previous pregnancy.
- Women who have a previous obstetric history of repeated miscarriages or unexplained stillbirths; or delivered a child with a congenital malformation.
- Women who have delivered a previous infant weighing more than 4.0 kg.

Risk factors for incipient diabetes and GDM

The gold standard for screening these women is the use of the 75-gram oral glucose tolerance test [oGTT]. The test involves taking three blood samples before and at subsequent hours after consuming a drink containing 75 grams of glucose (a form of sugar). By establishing a diagnosis of diabetes or IGT, good metabolic control can be achieved before embarking on a pregnancy thus reducing the risks of early pregnancy loss through a spontaneous miscarriage or the maldevelopment of the early embryo causing malformations. In the absence of pre-conceptional screening, the woman at risk in early pregnancy should be screened for hyperglycaemia as early as possible in the pregnancy. This screening usually involves performing a fasting blood glucose estimation, an HbA1c estimation, and ideally an oGTT.

Blood glucose	Non-pregnant		1st & early 2nd trimester	Late 2nd & 3rd trimester
	IGT	DM	DIP	GDM
• Fasting	≥6.1 mmol/l	≥7.0 mmol/l	≥7.0 mmol/l	≥5.1 mmol/l
• 1-hour				≥10.0 mmol/l
• 2-hours	≥7.8 mmol/l	≥11.1 mmol/l	≥11.1 mmol/l	≥8.5 mmol/l

Diagnostic criteria for the 75-gram oGTT

Gestational diabetes is one of the most common complications of pregnancy. It usually develops during the second half of pregnancy, when hormones interfere with the body's ability to use its natural insulin. Gestational diabetes does not have any particular risks to the mother, though it is associated with an increase in pregnancy-related hypertensive disease. It is very often symptomless, although some women may experience extreme thirst, hunger, or fatigue. Herein lies the danger since a pregnant woman with gestational diabetes is unaware that she is diabetic and does not seek attention. Gestational diabetes does affect the baby. Babies of all women with poorly controlled gestational diabetes are at increased risk of being of very high birth weights. This means that there may be more problems during delivery with an increased risk of damaging the child. After birth infants of women with gestational diabetes are more likely to suffer from breathing difficulties, low blood sugar levels and jaundice. Poorly controlled gestational diabetes also slightly increases the risk of delivering a dead baby. However, with improvements in medical care, stillbirth is rare. There are also long-term consequences for the GDM woman and her child. About 10 years after the pregnancy, about 67% of women who suffer from gestational diabetes develop diabetic problems particularly if they become obese. Babies of GDM women also may be at increased risk of developing obesity and diabetes as teens or young adults. Pregnancy can thus be seen as an opportunity to look into the future and assess the risks of subsequently developing diabetes.

It is therefore generally recommended that all women should be screened with a 75-gram oGTT at around 22-24 weeks of pregnancy to identify these women. The diagnostic criteria used at this stage of pregnancy needs to take cognisance of the normal physiological changes associated with the pregnancy state and therefore are different from those used in the non-pregnancy or first trimester criteria. Alternative to universal screening with an oGTT, the health carers may opt to screen women using a fasting blood glucose level and screen with an oGTT those women with a raised blood glucose level, or those who fall in a higher risk category, or those women who have clinical indicators of GDM during pregnancy.

- Women showing excessive weight gain during pregnancy.
- Women who have repeated fasting state glycosuria [glucose in urine].
- Women who have evidence of a large infant or increased liquor volume [polyhydramnios].
- Women with a family history of diabetes especially maternal and siblings.
- Women with elevated fasting blood glucose [>5.1 mmol/l], or elevated glucose 1 hour after meals [>8.0 mmol/l].

Clinical indicators suggesting GDM during pregnancy

Antenatal management: GDM and obese women are in the majority adequately managed with an appropriate dietary regimen suited to their day-to-day needs based on the woman's weight, lifestyle, and personal circumstances. The same dietary principles described for the woman with pre-pregnancy diabetes apply. The recommended diet for the GDM woman or obese is still based on the plate dietary plan method generally recommended for healthy eating. This healthy eating guide places emphasis to eat a greater proportion of foods such as complex carbohydrates (bread, pasta, rice, potatoes, and other cereals), mixed fruits and vegetables than protein foods (chicken, fish, legumes, lean red meat, eggs, nuts, and low-fat dairy products). All sugary and sweet products should be avoided at all costs. Frequent small meals may facilitate improved blood glucose control. Exercise remains an essential feature of maintaining the woman's wellbeing.

There are a few changes to be made to accommodate the increased nutritional needs for the developing child in utero. The expected total weight gain throughout pregnancy should be in the order of about 10-12kgs. This amount varies from woman-to-woman depending on the body weight and thus may be very much less in those who are overweight.

- An increased energy intake of about 200-300 calories a day is needed during the 2nd and 3rd trimesters only. This value varies depending on the physical activity levels between days and is the equivalent of about 2-3 slices of bread (50 grams each). These extra bread slices also provide the extra grams of proteins that are required during pregnancy.
- Meals should be split up throughout the day to about 3 meals a day. If blood sugar is difficult to control by eating three large meals a day, splitting daily food into 6 or 8 smaller ones, regularly spaced, and carefully planned maybe a better option.
- Increase the fibre and starch (bread, potatoes, cereals, rice, pasta) portion of every meal. Cut down on fatty foods.
- Increase the fruit and vegetables portions to at least 5 portions day.

Nutritional changes needed during pregnancy

Most women can control their blood sugar levels with diet alone. However, if blood sugar levels do not stabilise after two weeks with a controlled diet, pharmacological treatment utilizing oral hypoglycaemic agents and/or insulin injections may be needed daily for the remainder of the pregnancy. The introduction of pharmacological treatment is indicated when the fasting or pre-meal blood glucose values are persistently above 5.5 mmol/l. oral hypoglycaemic agents used during pregnancy include metformin and glibencamide. Insulin can be introduced as an alternative but is definitely indicated when the fasting or pre-meal blood glucose values are persistently above 7.0 mmol/l.

While the risks for a complicated pregnancy for women who develop gestational diabetes are much less than those for women who have diabetes before they became pregnant, it is to keep blood sugars in as normal a range as possible to help prevent the child from developing the short-term and long-term complications associated with exposure to intrauterine hyperglycaemia.

Management during labour: The requirements during labour of the GDM woman managed with diet or oral hypoglycaemics are obviously different from those of the insulin-dependent pregnant woman. The former group can be generally managed as normal women provided that the progress of labour is spontaneous and not prolonged. The oral hypoglycaemic agents should be avoided during labour while regular blood glucose monitoring is warranted throughout the labour process. Any undue rises or drops in blood glucose levels in the GDM woman in labour can be managed by the introduction of a glucose and insulin infusion pump regimen. When prolonged labour is anticipated, it is best to prophylactically manage these women with the same regimen as for the insulin-dependent diabetics.

Management after delivery: After delivery, the blood sugar levels of the GDM woman should return to normal. However, those GDM women who required insulin to manage their blood sugar levels should be rechecked with an oGTT two months after delivery to ensure that their metabolism has returned to normal. Those with severe gestational diabetes may have persistence of the disorder, albeit in a minor form, after the delivery.

The GDM women, and the overtly obese women, have been shown to develop frank carbohydrate intolerance later in life, reflecting their underlying insulin resistance status. All GDM women should therefore be encouraged to check their carbohydrate metabolism status annually to identify early the development of any impairment and thus institute timely metabolic and medical intervention. They should particularly reassess their metabolic status prior to embarking on another pregnancy. All these women should be further about the nutritional and physical activity measures they should adopt to prevent the development or the augmentation of obesity – another known risk factor for the development of Type 2 diabetes. Babies born to GDM and obese mothers also have a higher lifetime risk of obesity and of developing Type 2 diabetes. These children should be regularly screened during childhood to ensure that adequate measures are taken to reduce the risks of developing childhood obesity.

Complication Screening [1]

Diabetes is a complex disease that leads to serious complications due to (uncontrolled) elevated blood sugar (glucose) levels in your body. Diabetes complications can be prevented or delayed if you are on the lookout for symptoms and follow your doctor's advice while being compliant with medication. These complications can be divided into acute and chronic complications.

Acute diabetes complications

These complications can occur at any time and if left untreated may progress to chronic (long-term) complications. The acute complications can be classified into four:

a) *Hypos (hypoglycaemic episode)*: this occurs when the blood sugar (glucose) is too low. The person experiencing a hypo will feel very tired, dizzy, hungry, irritated, tearful, anxious, or moody, sweaty, and trembling. One may also experience lack of concentration or blurred vision and fast heart rate. Therefore, if you experience any of these symptoms, and you have a capillary blood glucose monitor easily accessible, check your blood glucose. Even if you do not have access to such monitor, it is recommended to consume sugary sweets or a sugary drink, followed by a carbohydrate snack such as a sandwich or a cereal bar. Hypos tend to happen if a meal is delayed or missed, if a lower portion of carbohydrates is ingested than usual, if extra exercise or physical activity is performed without consuming a carbohydrate snack, if taking too much medication or else if drinking alcohol.

b) *Hypers (hyperglycaemic episode)*: this occurs when the blood sugar (glucose) is too high. The commonest symptoms that are experiences in such a hyper state are: feeling very thirsty, weak, or tired, blurred vision, increased urination and losing weight. To

---

[1] Prepared by Dr. Sarah Cuschieri.

avoid such episodes, it is imperative to be compliant with the diabetes medication that is prescribed, avoid eating too much starchy or sugary foods, maintain a regular exercise regimen while losing weight if overweight, as well as try to avoid stressful periods.

c) *Hyperosmolar Hyperglycaemic State (HHS)*: this a life-threatening emergency that may occurs if suffering from type 2 diabetes. The common symptoms of HHS are experiencing severe thirst, nausea, dry skin, increased urination, disorientation that can progress to drowsiness and gradual loss of consciousness. HHS requires emergency admission to hospital for urgent treatment. To avoid experiencing HHS it is imperative to take the diabetes medication even if sick while monitoring the blood glucose level regularly. Make sure to contact your family doctor if the blood glucose levels are constantly high.

d) *Diabetic ketoacidosis (DKA)*: this a life-threatening emergency that may occurs if suffering from type 1 diabetes. The commonest symptoms are feeling tired and sleepy, feeling very thirsty, increased urination, experiencing confusion, blurred vision, stomach pain and feeling sick. Having sweet / fruit smelling breath and passing out. It is important that individuals with type 1 diabetes monitor their blood glucose levels regularly and to speak immediately to their family doctor on noticing high blood glucose levels.

Chronic diabetes complications

Individuals with long standing diabetes are more prone to develop chronic complications over time, especially those with uncontrolled blood glucose levels. Chronic complications develop gradually and can affect different bodily organs resulting in various problems.

a) *Heart attack and stroke*: long standing high blood glucose levels damage the blood vessels. Over a period this can result in the occlusion of the main arterial blood flow to the heart leading to a heart attack. If the arterial blood flow to be brain is compromised, then a stroke can occur.

100

b) *Kidney problems (nephropathy)*: high blood glucose in association with high blood pressure (hypertension) can overtime damage the kidneys. The kidney normal function of clearing of waste products would be compromised resulting in kidney disease.

c) *Nerve damage (neuropathy)*: one of the complications of high glucose levels is nerve damage that temper nerve messages from being transmitted between organs. This leads to problems with hearing, feeling, and moving.

d) *Eye problems (retinopathy)*: in some individuals the high glucose levels affect the eyesight. If a regular eye screening test is undertaken, this can be picked up early and treated with the prevention of loss of eyesight.

e) *Foot problems*: the occurrence of nerve and blood vessel damage due to high blood glucose can result in foot problems because of lack of sensation and impaired healing of sores and cuts that may have been sustained in the foot. This can lead to serious foot problems requiring amputation.

f) *Gum disease*: high blood glucose levels can lead to high sugar in saliva which in turn can result in gum disease.

g) *Sexual problems*: the restricted blood flow due to damaged blood vessels as a secondary effect of high blood glucose can lead to various problems to the sexual organs in both females and males.

How to avoid getting complications?
The key to preventing complications is to monitor your blood glucose, be compliant with the prescribed medication and visit your family doctor regularly for check-ups. Yearly physical and routine eye check-ups should also be scheduled and attended. These yearly check-ups are important as the doctor will screen for the development of potential chronic diabetes complications. Dental check-ups should also be scheduled at least twice a year.

Maintaining a healthy lifestyle by eating a balanced diet and being physically active forms part of the diabetes management plan that you should follow.

Smoking should be avoided, as smoking induces the risk of diabetes complications such as the reduction of blood flow to the feet, worsening blood glucose control, increase the susceptibility to heart disease, stroke, nerve damage, eye disease, kidney damage as well as premature death.

Alcohol should be consumed moderately and ideally with food. Alcohol can lead to both high and low blood glucose levels, dependent on the quantity consumed and whether food had been eaten or not.

As part of the diabetes management plan, it is important that you and your doctor keep track of your blood pressure and cholesterol levels. Both high blood pressure and high cholesterol levels can damage your blood vessels or occlude them, resulting in heart attacks and strokes.

The feet should be regularly inspected for any redness, blisters, sores, swelling or calluses. Daily washing of your feet should be done using lukewarm water while avoiding prolonged soaking of feet, as this predisposes to dry skin. The feet should be dried gently, and moisturising creams applied, although this should be avoided between toes. It is imperative not to walk barefoot and if you observe any foot problem to consult your doctor immediately.

Contributor biographies

Dr. Mario J. Cachia – Consultant Physician and Endocrinologist within the Malta Healthcare Services at Mater Dei University Hospital, Malta; Visiting Senior Lecturer in Medicine within the Faculty of Medicine & Surgery of the University of Malta; Lead Clinician at the Gender Wellbeing Clinic which looks after clients' various aspects of transgender care.

Dr. Mario Caruana Grech Perry –Registered Dietitian in the public and private healthcare sectors in Malta; Lecturer within the Department of Food Sciences and Nutrition at the Faculty of Health Sciences, University of Malta. Doctoral thesis: *The effect of dietary components (polyphenols) on protein misfolding in neurodegenerative diseases and diabetes* [2011].

Dr. Claire Copperstone – Registered pharmacist and nutritionist; Senior Lecturer in Human Nutrition within the Department of Food Sciences and Nutrition at the Faculty of Health Sciences, University of Malta; past-Member [2016-2017] of the Maltese Presidency working group on obesity, member of the British Nutrition Society and Malta contact for the World Obesity Federation. Doctoral thesis: *A novel dietary assessment tool and a feasibility study to improve sugar and water consumption in Maltese schoolchildren* [2013].

Dr. Johann Craus – Consultant Obstetrician-Gynaecologist within the Malta Healthcare Services managing the Diabetic Pregnancy Joint Clinic at Mater Dei University Hospital, Malta; Visiting Senior Lecturer in Obstetrics-Gynaecology within the Faculty of Medicine & Surgery of the University of Malta. Doctoral thesis: *Genetics and inflammatory markers for gestational diabetes mellitus* [2016].

Dr. Sarah Cuschieri – Physician with an interest in Endocrinology and Public Health; Lecturer within the Faculty of Medicine & Surgery of the University of Malta; Co-founder and president of the Malta Obesity Association which serves as an NGO targeting obesity in Malta; Member of the Faculty of Public Health of the United Kingdom; Dame of the

Grand Priory of the Maltese Islands of the Military & Hospitaller Order of St Lazarus of Jerusalem. Doctoral thesis: *Burden of Diabetes Mellitus Type 2, dysglycaemia and their co-determinants in the adult population of Malta* [2019].

Ms. Moira Grixti – Senior Practice Nurse in Diabetes managing the Diabetes Education Unit at Mater Dei University Hospital, Malta; visiting lecturer at the Faculties of Medicine and Surgery and of Health Sciences of the University of Malta; Vice-President of the Maltese Diabetes Association. Master thesis: *A Service Development Project to Assess Incident Hypoglycaemia and Associated Care Delivery Factors In Hospitalized Patients with Diabetes* [2019].

Prof. Charles Savona-Ventura – Consultant Obstetrician-Gynaecologist (retired) within the Malta Healthcare Services managing the Diabetic Pregnancy Joint Clinic at Mater Dei University Hospital, Malta; Head and Professor of the Obstetrics-Gynaecology Department within the Faculty of Medicine & Surgery and Director for the Centre for Traditional Chinese Medicine of the University of Malta; Visiting Professor to Shanghai University for TCM; International Grand Hospitaller & Grand Prior of the Maltese Islands of the Military & Hospitaller Order of St Lazarus of Jerusalem. Doctoral thesis: *The significance of GIGT in the Maltese population* [1996].

Ms. Stephanie Savona-Ventura – Healthcare psychologist within the Malta Healthcare Services responsible for providing psychological services to paediatric Type 1 diabetics and grossly obese individuals presenting for bariatric surgery at Mater Dei University Hospital, Malta; Visiting lecturer within the Faculty of Medicine & Surgery and the Faculty for Social Wellbeing of the University of Malta. Master thesis: *Changes in parental control and parenting styles across three generations and their impact on dietary habits in Malta* [2012]. Currently reading for a doctoral degree researching psychological issues in paediatric Type 1 diabetics.

Prof. Josanne Vassallo – Consultant Physician and Endocrinologist within the Malta Healthcare Services at Mater Dei University Hospital, Malta; Professor of Medicine within the Faculty of Medicine & Surgery of the University of Malta. Member of a number of European and American Endocrine and Diabetes Societies and served from as past-President [2013-

2017] of the Mediterranean Group for the Study of Diabetes with the remit of fostering research and disseminating knowledge regarding Diabetes in the Mediterranean. Doctoral thesis: *Paracrine regulation of testicular function: the role of epidermal growth factor and insulin-like growth factor-I in spermatogenesis* [1991].

Dr. Sandro Vella – Consultant Physician, Diabetologist and Endocrinologist within the Malta Healthcare Services at Mater Dei University Hospital, Malta; Visiting Senior Lecturer in Medicine within the Faculty of Medicine & Surgery of the University of Malta. Master thesis: *Thyroid dysfunction in a Maltese type 2 diabetes population* [2008]; Doctoral thesis: *Pharmacological modulation of insulin resistance: benefits and harms* [2013].

www.ingramcontent.com/pod-product-compliance
Lightning Source LLC
Chambersburg PA
CBHW070204290526
45789CB00002B/900